EDI
A Guide to Electronic Data Interchange and Electronic Commerce Applications in the Healthcare Industry

EDI

A Guide to Electronic Data Interchange and Electronic Commerce Applications in the Healthcare Industry

James J. Moynihan

Marcia L. McLure, Ph.D.

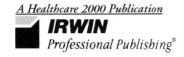

A Healthcare 2000 Publication
IRWIN
Professional Publishing®

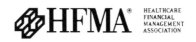

HFMA®   HEALTHCARE
         FINANCIAL
         MANAGEMENT
         ASSOCIATION

Irwin Book Team

Editor:	Kris Rynne
Project editor:	Amy E. Lund
Production supervisor:	Lara Feinberg
Assistant manager, desktop services:	Jon Christopher
Interior designer:	Matthew Baldwin
Jacket designer:	Palmer Design Associates
Compositor:	Electronic Publishing Services, Inc.
Typeface:	11/13 Palatino
Printer:	Braun-Brumfield

Library of Congress Cataloging-in-Publication Data

Moynihan, James J.
    EDI: a guide for the health professional / James J. Moynihan.
      p.   cm.
    Previously published: Chicago, Ill. : Probus Co., 1993.
    Includes index.
    ISBN 1-55738-624-2
    1. Electronic data interchange.   2. Health facilities—Business management.   I. Title
    RA971.3.M68   1996
    362.1'068'1—dc20   95–20229

This book is dedicated to the volunteers in healthcare and insurance standards organizations whose countless hours of hard work have laid the foundation for EDI in Health Care.

Contents

Chapter Nine
ORGANIZING FOR EDI 125

Chapter Ten
FINANCIAL EDI 135

Preface

EDI: A Guide to Electronic Data Interchange and Electronic Commerce Applications in the Healthcare Industry explores applications of electronic data interchange (EDI) and electronic commerce for the healthcare industry. The focus of the book is on the use of electronic networks that can be used to link participants in the healthcare industry. These networks are used to exchange information that would traditionally be exchanged on paper through the mail. Networks facilitate the paperless exchange of information between different organizations. This is a different concept from the so-called paperless office, in which electronic mail, imaging, and other technologies are used to eliminate paper used within an organization. The term *electronic commerce* is used to describe paperless exchanges between different organizations. Electronic commerce has a multitude of applications. It includes intercorporate electronic mail, facsimile machines, and magnetic card readers. It may include wireless communications and other technologies as they become available.

EDI places a particular focus on a subset of electronic commerce called electronic data interchange (EDI). EDI allows transactions to be exchanged between the computer of one organization and the computer of another organization without human intervention. EDI is the least costly, most effective way to exchange information that does not need to be reviewed by humans. EDI may not be technologically the most exciting aspect of electronic commerce, but the technology employed embodies the business discipline of "standardized" business processes. All the technology in the world cannot automate a Tower of Babel in which industry participants do not support standards.

The healthcare system in the United States is said to encompass 15 percent of the Gross Domestic Product and healthcare costs are estimated to exceed $1 trillion. The application of electronic commerce technologies to this industry presents an enormous opportunity to eliminate countless inefficient paper-based transactions. Major progress has been made. Standards-based EDI, for example, was limited solely to the exchange of purchase orders and related documents in 1990. Electronic claims submission and electronic claims payment grew exponentially during the early 1990s. By the mid-1990s standards-based EDI for claims processing was the official policy of the Health Care Financing Administration and most health insurance organizations. In addition to concrete implementations, the vision of a networked healthcare system became the subject of media attention and a key component of healthcare reform. Consensus grew about the potential applications that included

- Automated claims processing that could substantially reduce administrative costs.
- Electronic exchange of portions of an electronic patient record to cut administrative costs and improve the clinical quality of care provided.
- The capability that would enable researchers to tap into electronic clinical data in many locations to uncover outcomes assessment data that could transform the way in which medicine is delivered.
- The vision of a networked healthcare system with all participants linked to exchange data is generally referred to as the *community healthcare information network (CHIN)*. Projects to create CHINs are occurring throughout the country and provide a variety of experiments to move the industry to a networked future.

Getting to a totally electronic exchange of all the crucial documents in the healthcare industry will take time. The long-range vision is attractive, but the progress will have to take place one step at a time. Soon many providers will automate both accounts receivable and procurement processing. Benefit administrators will electronically link to employers for enrollment data and with providers for claims processing. Benefit administrators and providers will also adapt EDI to new ways of organizing the healthcare delivery system under managed care. These challenges and the implementation of clinical exchanges will provide a full agenda for the healthcare industry.

These changes in the way healthcare information is managed will require a commitment from senior management, not just more resources for the information systems department. EDI is not a *systems* initiative but a *managerial* one. From a systems standpoint, EDI is not technologically challenging, and the cost of EDI software is an inconsequential portion of the typical systems budget. Although using EDI is not technically difficult, its implementation is not easy. EDI is complex from a managerial standpoint because it fundamentally changes the jobs people are expected to perform and the ways in which an organization is structured. Managers must develop the strategy to link electronically with "trading partners" and manage the conversion from the use of paper documents to their electronic replacements.

If the healthcare industry is as successful in the use of EDI as other industries have been, it will tap underused assets of both capital and personnel. Providers will do a better job of fulfilling their mission with fewer resources while providing a more responsive service and a better quality of care. Benefit administrators will provide better customer service with lower costs. In short, by using EDI, the industry can raise the standards of the healthcare services it provides while substantially lowering the administrative costs involved.

James J. Moynihan
Marcia L. McLure, Ph.D.

EDI
A Guide to Electronic Data
Interchange and Electronic
Commerce Applications in
the Healthcare Industry

I

OVERVIEW OF EDI

Chapter One

Features and Benefits of EDI

WHAT IS EDI?

In most organizations paperwork abounds for routine repetitive business transactions. Many businesses have begun to eliminate some of this paperwork by computerization. For example, accounting transactions were once recorded on ledger cards, but in most organizations ledger cards have been replaced by computers. Most automation however, has been applied only to information used within an organization. The standard operating procedure for sending information to other organizations is to print and mail paper documents. Every day, across the United States, the information on millions of computer-generated documents is keyed into other computers, as Figure 1–1 illustrates. Electronic data interchange (EDI) radically changes that process.

Electronic data interchange is the transmission, via a telecommunications network, of information from the computer system of one organization to the computer system of another. EDI is formally defined as the exchange of computer processable data in a standard format without human intervention.

The use of EDI eliminates many paper documents. It has proven to be of great benefit in many industries and in many countries around the world. This does not imply that there is anything inherently wrong with using paper, nor is there anything inherently inefficient about the use of paper for presenting information (as in this book). It is realistic to expect that paper documents will continue to be used for some purposes in the foreseeable future. Fundamentally, EDI does not seek to eliminate paper so much as paperwork.

FIGURE 1–1

Much of the information that becomes computer input is output from other computers.

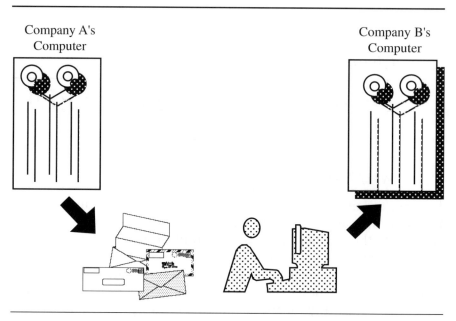

Because the healthcare industry in the United States processes an immense amount of paperwork, the time is ripe for applying EDI to all healthcare administrative processes. EDI has already been implemented successfully in many industries, so little new technology is required to apply EDI principles to healthcare. What is most required is the willingness of participants in the healthcare industry to explore the ways in which EDI could transform their work processes.

WHAT CAN EDI DO?

Electronic data interchange is a tool that can help organizations in the healthcare industry in the following ways:

- Eliminate unnecessary paperwork
- Reduce the time it takes to do a job

- Forge better working relationships with trading partners
- Introduce improved business methods

Eliminating Unnecessary Paperwork

EDI provides a solution for managers who seek to work faster and better with fewer resources. Paperwork can be slashed when a standard paper form exchanged between two organizations, such as a claim or a purchase order, can be transmitted electronically. Additional paperwork can be eliminated when all the forms exchanged in a business process are automated. Automating a whole series of paper exchanges has produced some of the most dramatic success stories.

The use of EDI in other industries for the entire procurement process is one of the most common and fully documented applications of EDI. Resulting cost savings can be dramatic. Pacific Bell, for example, estimated its total cost of processing paper-based procurement documents at about $73 per order.[1] By using EDI to replace all the paper documents exchanged with vendors, the cost of procurement was lowered to less than $4 per order. These large savings were obtained by using electronic purchase orders, electronic advance shipping notices, barcoding of shipments, electronic invoices, and electronic vendor payments. Savings also came from internal software enhancements that allowed the information that was sent electronically to be integrated with existing application programs, such as accounts payable and materials management. Comparable economies have been reported by companies in a variety of manufacturing and distribution industries.

The benefits achieved by many organizations in automating the procurement process can be matched by trading partners in the healthcare industry. In the claims process, EDI can be used from the first eligibility inquiry about a patient through the final claim payment. Automation of this process will result in even greater

---

[1] Pacific Bell's case was described by Mary Olivias, EDI product manager, procurement systems, in a presentation to the Southern California EDI Roundtable on May 31, 1991.
Author's additional note: Such large cost reductions usually come from the use of EDI and some reengineering of the underlying process.

benefits than automation of procurement. Various industry estimates that combine savings for both providers and claims payers have developed estimates of savings that range from $10 billion to $40 billion if widespread implementation is achieved. The Workgroup on EDI (WEDI), a consortium of provider and payer organizations interested in EDI, developed the first industry-wide estimates of savings from EDI in the claims process. WEDI's October 1993 report projected net savings of $42.3 billion during a six-year implementation. Providers were projected to save $26.1 billion, payers would save $9.4 billion, and employers would save $6.8 billion. While other studies have been conducted which produced lower savings estimates there is substantial consensus that EDI can save billions of dollars when implemented for claims processing.

Shortening the Cycle Time

Although the use of EDI can dramatically cut transaction costs, some of the most avid supporters of EDI are more concerned with the benefits of faster transaction processing. By eliminating barriers to the timely and accurate transfer of information, EDI allows greater responsiveness to customer needs and faster responses to markets. In many competitive industries, timely responses to the market are essential.

For example, in the retail industry, EDI is a fundamental feature of "quick response" techniques to meet consumer demand. Successful retailers have capitalized on the latest trends in fashion by providing garment manufacturers with information captured by point-of-sale terminals in stores. As a result, the supply of materials is matched to consumer demand. In manufacturing and distribution businesses, successful organizations are also using EDI to shorten the business cycle.

Speeding up the business process is crucial for participants in the healthcare industry as well. For example,

- What does it mean to an insurance company if employers update their list of enrolled lives daily rather than monthly? It means employers get an accurate bill and claims are not paid for ineligible claimants.

FIGURE 1–2
The manufacturing timeline. EDI can shrink the timeline, also known as a **business cycle,** *in manufacturing and many other healthcare industry processes.*

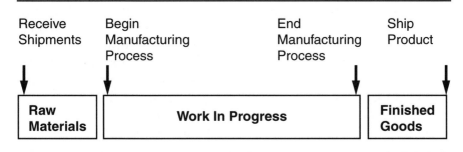

- What does it mean to a hospital if requests for supplies are not sent in a timely fashion to the correct supplier, or if physicians cannot get laboratory results quickly? Doing these tasks speedily results in better medicine and better customer service.

One method of analysis is widely used to measure such performance: the transaction timeline. Transaction timelines can be applied to an entire business process in any industry, such as the manufacturing one shown in Figure 1–2. The transaction timeline can also be used to portray subsections of a business transaction, such as the timeline for accounts receivable collection, which may be expressed in days, or for hospital admission processing, which may be expressed in minutes. For the provider the transaction timelines for the procurement and claims processes determine the funds tied up in inventory and accounts receivable. Managed care organizations have a vital interest in managing the utilization review timeline. The efficiency of these processes determines how many people are employed in financial administration.

Plotting a transaction timeline is the first step in an engineering approach to cost reduction. The business process under review is measured, the time it takes to complete the job determined, and the transactions in the process required to complete the job are identified. EDI is a tool to streamline the process and shorten the transaction timeline.

In an era of downsizing, rightsizing, and competitive pressure, intelligent cost management is necessary. As financial pressures on organizations intensify, managers are asked to slash their budgets. That requires analysis of the tasks employees perform and how those tasks can be changed to shorten the transaction timeline. Bureaucrats merely manipulate budgets, but good managers design the work flows to shorten the tasks' completion time.[2] It makes little sense to eliminate workers without eliminating work. The computer-to-computer exchange of information eliminates the work and direct costs of transaction processing. When EDI shortens the transaction timeline it also lowers the cash investment in inventory and receivables. By cutting transaction costs and capital tied up in the business EDI reduces the largest components of cost.

Forging Links with Trading Partners

Many organizations have invested a great deal in computer systems to automate information management. The different emphasis of EDI is of automating information sent *between* organizations, not just information used internally. Many EDI users report that the gains from improvements in business techniques with external organizations may be greater than the improvements available internally. The best practices of America's corporations in recent years have shown that suppliers and vendors play a crucial role in the production of a high-quality product. Adversarial relationships between buyers and vendors have proven to be counterproductive. The better approach is to view all the organizations with which vital information is exchanged as trading partners.

For those that have pursued this approach, electronic links with trading partners have become essential business procedures. In manufacturing, EDI makes "just-in-time" inventory management possible through the immediate electronic transfer of inventory requirements. The grocery industry has widely adopted EDI and related barcoding to transform the checkout process at most supermarkets. These applications of EDI are well documented and fully

---

[2] For an excellent discussion of process management and cost reduction, see H. Thomas Johnson and Robert S. Kaplan, *Relevance Lost: The Rise and Fall of Management Accounting* (Boston: Harvard Business School Press, 1987).

FIGURE 1–3

Major trading partners such as these exchange information and funds on a repetitive basis that can be automated using EDI.

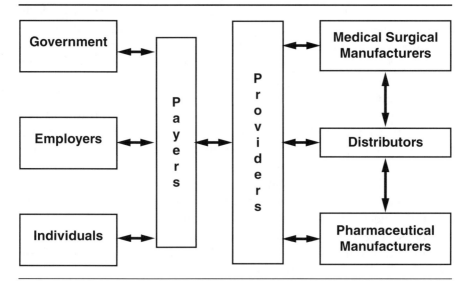

described in other books and articles.[3] The trading partner approach views the buyer/vendor exchange of information and products as more than a bidding process to arrive at the lowest bid price. Companies that obtain higher quality and lower costs through partnerships with their suppliers can increase value to the consumer. The same logic applies to participants in the healthcare industry. Figure 1–3 diagrams some major trading partner relationships for the healthcare industry.

The underlying principles adopted by other industries to cut product costs through trading partner linkages can be used in health care. Like the grocery industry, hospitals and their suppliers can use barcoding and EDI to slash costs. Just as the automobile industry has adopted "just-in-time" inventory management to change the logistics of dealing with its suppliers, hospitals can adopt variations on the practice known as "stockless purchasing."

---

[3] For a list of EDI resources, see Appendix A.

Technologies called "point of sale" in a retail store can be called "point of service" when providers initiate an eligibility inquiry for a patient using swipe card technology.

The benefits of working with, rather than against, trading partners can also be achieved by providers and claims payers. The administration of claims processing and medical reimbursement is a major component of the final cost of health care in the United States. In 1991, a *New England Journal of Medicine* article reported that 24 percent of the total cost of health care was attributable to the cost of administration.[4] EDI can lower these administrative costs. This may seem like a daunting task because of the size of the healthcare industry, yet the intolerably high costs of health care make greater efficiency a necessity.

The challenge to healthcare industry participants is to duplicate the success of EDI in other industries. Trading partners can forge not only electronic links but greater agreement about how to do business. The computer-to-computer information exchange is at the heart of the formal definition of EDI, but the spirit of EDI is best expressed when trading partners find better ways to do business.

Adopting Improved Business Methods

As well as automating current procedures, EDI enables its users to improve the way they do business. Each of the three examples that follow illustrates how the use of EDI improves operations.

Example 1: Using EDI eliminates the uncertainty of knowing whether a transmitted document arrived at its intended destination.

How often have you mailed a letter and wondered whether it arrived? That uncertainty is avoided in an electronic environment. Most EDI users send an acknowledgment of receipt back to the transmitting party. This is the electronic counterpart of sending registered return receipt mail but at a fraction of the cost and time. Confirmation that a message has been received can be followed by the acknowledgment that it has been processed by the appropriate

---

4 Steffie Woolhandler and David U. Himmelstein, "The Deteriorating Administrative Efficiency and the U.S. Health Care System," *New England Journal of Medicine* 324: 1253-58 (May 2, 1991).

application program of the receiver. Insurance companies can acknowledge receipts of claims, and distributors can acknowledge receipts of purchase orders. Providers have a greater certainty that claims will be paid and supplies will be delivered when acknowledgments are available from trading partners. This process is an improvement over most paper-based practices and eliminates the phone calls that inquire "Did you get the message?", "Was the information correct?", and "Did you process the transaction?"

Example 2: Using EDI forces users to focus on and improve the details of repetitive business transactions.

Organizations that begin to trade information electronically also begin to examine the information they exchange with an unprecedented focus on detail. This intense focus on how work is done is an important first step to converting from paper to electronic exchanges. The frequent result is that the analysis reveals correctable flaws in current procedures. The benefit is a substantial reduction in errors and a related improvement in performance. Why were these steps not taken before? Few organizations stop to closely review many of their mundane business procedures. Processing invoices and remittances, generating paper claim forms, and creating purchase orders are all part of payables and receivables practices that have been done in the same way for decades. Paper forms may change from time to time, but many are "homegrown" and are used without question. The transition from paper to electronic commerce presents an opportunity for creative managers to step back and ask fundamental questions about the business process.

Example 3: EDI users can upgrade internal procedures to the industry standard.

Although poor business practices can creep into any organization, they are more likely to develop in those areas where a department interacts with another organization. In internal departments, a "company policy" can standardize procedures, forms, and practices and bring order to an administrative process. In departments that deal with the outside world, employees must deal with paperwork in whatever form it comes their way from other companies. How many different formats of invoices and remittance advices must a hospital contend with?

Providers inflict the same problems on their trading partners. How do large distributors cope with various different purchase orders? How many differently formatted claim forms does a large insurance company have to process? When trading partners start to cooperate, they can avail themselves of EDI standards (see Chapter 2) that incorporate the experience of others who have been working on improving business procedures for years. EDI users have developed the means to get the right information to the right place at the right time.

EDI OPPORTUNITIES: RETHINKING THE WAY WE DO BUSINESS

EDI is a common sense idea that is relatively simple to understand and yet complex to implement. Technological developments such as easy-to-use telecommunications and inexpensive hardware and software have helped spread the use of EDI. The more important factor in the implementation of EDI, however, is the agreement among trading partners that EDI is the best way to do business. Opportunities to use EDI have been grasped by organizations willing to rethink the way they do business. Unchallenged assumptions about how business is done may be the greatest roadblock to the success of EDI. Managers in the healthcare industry must adopt three new assumptions about how they will do business in the future.

Assumption 1: EDI , Not Keying, Is the Standard Operating Procedure for Data Capture

Most of us have spent our lives dealing with paper and not with "computer-processable data" and so doing business electronically requires exploration of new territories. Think about how most information traditionally gets into computers. During the last 10 years, the experience most people have had with computers has been one of sitting in front of a screen and typing in information in response to prompts appearing on the screen. Before the 1980s, it was common for larger mini- or mainframe computers to be used with many "dumb" terminals linked to the central computer. The mindset of using "our" terminals to get data into "our" computer still dominates the thinking within many companies.

Many hospitals use such terminals given to them by their fiscal intermediaries to enter claim data. They may also use different terminals provided by their distributors to enter purchase orders. Many insurance companies provide their employer customers with terminals to change or look up current eligibility information.

The assumption that information is "normally" exchanged through rekeying data from documents into another computer in an information chain is one of the largest impediments to computer-to-computer exchanges of information.

Software vendors will continue to develop systems predicated on repetitive data entry until their customers ask for automated entry capabilities. This is not a technical issue but an example of the importance of habits—of accepted ways of doing business that have become outmoded.

Assumption 2: EDI Is the Standard Operating Procedure for Doing Business Electronically; Tapes, Faxes, and E-mails Have Their Uses but Are Not EDI

To achieve maximum efficiency, electronic transmissions should be received and processed without human intervention. Computers can receive information through batch transfers. Batch transfers have historically been done using magnetic tapes. Information from one computer is recorded onto a magnetic tape and the tape is shipped to be mounted and read by the receiving computer. Sometimes called "tape-to-tape" transfer, this has been an accepted procedure in health care for many years. Also known as *electronic media claims (EMC)*, tape-to-tape transfers are still used by many companies in the healthcare insurance industry. EMC is actively promoted by claims payers that can accept electronic claims on tapes and diskettes of various sizes and formats. Although this is a form of electronic commerce, it requires human intervention, which adds cost and the potential for error to the information exchange. Tapes and diskettes must be shipped and mounted by the recipient. In the process, they may become corrupted or lost.

Telecommunications is the preferred medium for EDI, because there is no handling requirement for successful transmission. Telecommunications of claims among providers and payers is becoming more widespread. Although telecommunications is preferable for EDI, all telecommunicated messages are not EDI. Electronic mail and fax transmissions, for example, lack an essential feature: the information they carry is not computer-processable. Data from fax transmissions must be reentered into a computer just as if the document had arrived in the mail. Electronic mail messages must be read by the receiver, and because they consist of freeform text, they cannot be processed by a computer program at the receiving organization. EDI messages can be processed by a computer on receipt because they are transmitted in a standardized format. Fax and E-mail exchanges have a vital role to play in the exchange of business information but managers must recognize that EDI is preferable for most repetitive business transactions.

Assumption 3: Standard EDI Formats Are Vastly Superior to Nonstandard Formats

Standard formats are needed for more widespread electronic transmission of information. The need for consistent, standard formats can be illustrated by comparing electronic claims management with paper claim forms. Forms are marvelous ways to organize information on paper so that readers can find what they need in a "standardized" position. Each box is designed with enough blank space to hold the expected amount of information. Computer file formats for batch transfers are designed similarly. As Figure 1–4 shows, if a paper form were to be cut into thin strips along the bottom edge of each row of boxes and laid end to end, the result would look very similar to the way in which the specifications of a computer tape format are portrayed.

A sequence of information taken from the computer is called a *file*, and the specifications for its "boxes" are called the *file format*. If information from a computer is put on tape, it must be in the file format required by the receiving computer. The problem with these formats is that only a small difference between them—say, a specification that the space allocated for street address information

FIGURE 1–4

We are familiar with paper forms, and computer file formats are their electronic equivalents. The key to EDI is the use of standard formats.

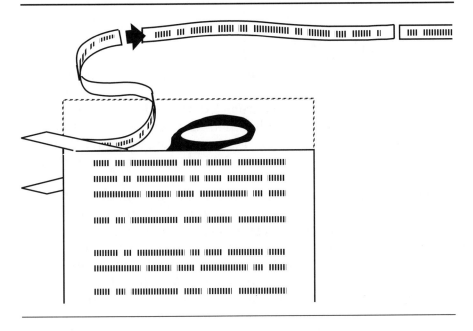

is 90 characters long instead of 88—can make one file format incompatible with another.

For example, consider the HCFA 1500 claim form, the most frequently used standard paper claim form for outpatient medical services. Although different claim payers may all agree about the information to list on the HCFA 1500, they may each require different proprietary formats designed to fit their particular needs. There are hundreds of electronic file formats for the electronic equivalents of the HCFA 1500 paper form and hundreds more for the inpatient claim form, the UB92. It is prohibitively expensive for providers to send claims electronically to different payers without payer support for format standards. There is an obvious need for an industry-wide standard format for the electronic claims process. (The issue of standards is discussed in greater detail in

Chapter 2.) The progress of EDI is hindered whenever trading partners fail to support standard formats. Managers must realize that support of EDI format standards is crucial.

THE FUTURE OF EDI

Healthcare industry participants have the benefit of learning from a decade of other industries' experiences with EDI applications. The success stories are well chronicled and, with a little work, the reasons for failures can be identified. Both successes and failures may help to answer the usual questions asked about the future of EDI: "Will it become widely used?" and "How can my institution benefit?"

Whether EDI is widely adopted is not a technological issue. Some industries may choose not to adopt a common electronic format because they have no desire to standardize the way business is conducted. Even if there is a desire to have a standard and the format is agreed on, mutual agreement about the information to be exchanged may be difficult to achieve. Whether EDI is widely used is primarily an issue of improved business practices with a dash of politics. Industry leaders must be willing to reach agreement about standards. When there have been no standards initiatives, there has frequently been no leadership.

During the 1980s the founders and members of the Health Industry Business Communications Council (HIBCC) exhibited the leadership needed to make EDI a reality for purchasing applications. During the early 1990s the efforts of hundreds of individuals from payer, provider, and government agency organizations created EDI standards for claims applications. The widespread use of insurance applications now appears to be inevitable. Because EDI standards have been embraced by such major institutions as the federal government, major commercial insurance companies, and Blue Cross Blue Shield organizations, they will be in widespread use by the late 1990s. The pace of change will be too slow for some organizations and too fast for others.

ADVANTAGES OF EDI REVISITED

To return to the first issue this chapter raised, how will organizations in the healthcare industry benefit from EDI? There are companies that use EDI and enjoy no real benefits, in large part because they were forced into participation. For example, some large companies stipulate to smaller vendors that use of EDI is required to process purchase orders. Rather than lose such major accounts, the smaller businesses install EDI software to receive the purchase orders and promptly print them. This form of EDI installation is not uncommon, and it is an expensive way to get the mail.

The failure of EDI in any application is usually a failure to achieve the potential expected. The benefits are limited because the usage is limited. This situation can occur when only a few trading partners make the transition from paper to EDI, or only a few of the many potential transactions in a business process are automated. In a similar fashion, some organizations will fail to reap the full benefits of EDI.

Far greater benefits are available to those who view EDI as a fundamental part of doing business in all departments. Farsighted providers recognize that their success depends on their ability to work with suppliers, payers, and others as trading partners with whom they can build relationships. Benefit administrators and insurance companies will use EDI to connect with employers and providers to offer higher levels of service at a lower cost. EDI can be a fundamental feature of the key relationships in the healthcare industry,

Developing and implementing EDI can create tremendous opportunities for change. When we change the way we do business, we reengineer our organizations to be more effective. This is why EDI starts out sounding like a mundane, low-technology process of transferring computer data but ends up being an exciting management strategy. EDI is not a technology; EDI is a better way of doing business that can benefit the healthcare industry.

Chapter Two

Standards and the Standards-Setting Process

The reason most people do not know much about standards is that society has already reached consensus on many standardization issues. We unthinkingly accept those standards that exist and only become aware of their importance when they do not exist. Standards are like the definition of salt given by a child: "Salt is the stuff in food that you know about when it isn't there." Standards play a vital role in our society, but when they function well they are virtually invisible. When you buy a light bulb, do you worry about what size socket is in your house? No, because almost all light bulbs and sockets conform to a single standard. You can pick up a telephone and call virtually anywhere in the world, and, despite the many different suppliers of telecommunication service, the systems are compatible enough for your call to go through. Healthcare providers become aware of standards when they lack them for the transactions that are important to the way in which payers and providers exchange information.

It is often assumed that standards are set by the government or by the marketplace and that there is little anyone can do to affect the outcome of the standards-setting process or to accelerate the acceptance of standards. The healthcare industry leadership must realize that the creation and support of standards are important business issues. The use of format standards and EDI software that supports those standards vastly simplifies the problems of interorganizational data exchange. Many healthcare providers use EDI software and national EDI standards for material management applications but not for the insurance-related transactions that make up the bulk of their revenues. To a large degree, this has been because, until recently, there were no EDI standards for the relevant documents, such as the claim and the claim payment/ remittance advice. Standards are now available for these and other healthcare insurance transactions. Because this is an important issue, it is worth reviewing the EDI standards development process. This is best done by first addressing the larger issue of standards creation.

HOW STANDARDS ARE DEVELOPED

Standards have been developed for a multitude of applications, from the nineteenth century's need for standardized railroad gauges to a host of telecommunications standards in the late twentieth century. Some efforts at standardization worked well and were implemented quickly; others resulted in major differences of opinion that were not reconciled for decades.

ANSI

In many countries governments decree standards through central bureaucracies. The United States, however, uses a voluntary national standards system. Since 1918, when it was chartered by Congress, the American National Standards Institute (ANSI) has had the responsibility for monitoring the creation of American national standards. The ANSI organization does not *make* the standards. It promulgates a consensus-based process with procedures to ensure fair and equitable standards creation. ANSI occupies the high ground of being the only organization through which a standard can become an official American national standard. Nonetheless, there are important healthcare standards in use that were not originally developed under the auspices of ANSI.

The ANSI consensus process is an important aspect of how standards are created. There can be no standard if a significant minority objects. Change is accommodated as the business case develops. New needs result in the creation of new standards-creating bodies under the ANSI umbrella. There are more than 10,000 ANSI standards that cover a multitude of areas. The ones that are relevant for this book are ANSI standards for EDI.

Precursors to ANSI's EDI Standards

The ANSI organization responsible for EDI standards was chartered in 1979. The movement to EDI can be traced back much earlier, however. The realization that it makes more sense to exchange standardized business documents electronically is not a new insight. Some of the pioneers in the field of EDI cite the 1948 Berlin airlift as the catalyst that directed logistics experts toward reducing the paperwork that impeded the rapid movement of goods. For example, the railroad industry saw the need to exchange information about the location of boxcars that were owned by one company but on the tracks of another.

Standards were developed to exchange such information in the 1950s. More than 30 years ago some companies were trying to use the principles of EDI by exchanging boxes of computer punch cards. In some industries, major companies encouraged their vendors to link with them electronically. In retailing, such giants as Sears Roebuck and Kmart each developed electronic links with their vendors. The linkages developed by dominant companies such as Sears and Kmart are classified as *proprietary standards.* In the healthcare industry a similar linkage using a proprietary standard was pioneered by the American Hospital Supply Corporation, whose ASAP system remains in use by many hospitals to order supplies.

The development of *industry-specific standards* was a natural next step in many industries. For example, the vendor that shipped to Sears might also deal with Kmart, Wal-Mart, and other retailers. With proprietary systems, that vendor might have several different terminals in operation to communicate with various customers. The 1970s saw parallel movements in different industries toward industry standards and away from proprietary systems. The property and casualty industry developed ACORD standards, the grocery industry created the UCS standards, and the transportation industry created the TDCC standards.[1]

---

[1] In health care during this period, an industry-specific claim form was developed, although not an electronic document. Most hospital providers are aware of the National Uniform Billing Committee sponsored by the American Hospital Association. The NUBC has representation from government and private sector payers as well as hospital providers. The NUBC has maintained the Uniform Bill and released new versions from time to time.

Although the development of industry-specific standards was logical, it became clear as time went on that industry-specific standards created new problems. For example, if a railroad carrier handles a shipment of grocery goods, should it communicate with the shipper using the grocery standards or the transportation standards? The solution to this kind of situation was to create a *cross-industry standard*.

ASC X12

In 1979, the oldest industry-specific standards organization, the Transportation Data Coordinating Committee, together with the Credit Research Foundation applied to ANSI to approve the creation of a standards group that would be responsible for cross-industry EDI standards. The resulting ANSI committee charged with that responsibility is the ANSI Accredited Standards Committee (ASC) X12. The work of ASC X12 is conducted primarily by a series of subcommittees and task groups whose major function is developing new EDI standards and maintaining existing standards.

During the 1980s, many corporations that had supported proprietary standards migrated to the emerging X12 standards. Industry associations that had developed their own standards moved to incorporate their needs into the X12 standards. The X12 mission is not one that involves reinventing or revising the data in standards developed by industry associations. There is a strong preference to have industry-specific code lists maintained separately from X12 and incorporated by reference. A large number of external code sources are already listed, and they have just been joined by codes familiar to healthcare providers (such as ICD codes and CPT/HCPCS codes). There is a high return from this limited mission. Incredible amounts of waste can be eliminated when one standard electronic format replaces the information normally found on a variety of different but equivalent formats. One recent book about EDI contained an estimate that as much as 25 percent of all computer programs in existence were written to reformat data from one file format to another.[2]

---

[2] Paul Kimberly, *Electronic Data Interchange* (New York: McGraw-Hill, 1991), p. 9.

Such waste may not be visible to managers in the healthcare industry because business processes have remained unchanged for many years. Managers have to stress within their organizations that adherence to doing business "up to the standards" must become the rule, not the exception. Managers must realize that these trends are inevitable in health care, as well as in many other sectors of the economy.

The challenge for standardization in health care is significant. In order to do business electronically, trading partners need to agree to support standard data content in business exchanges and agree to the EDI format standards. The healthcare industry has an advantage over many other industries because of the tradition of a standard paper claim form. Consider how difficult the challenge was facing other industries with thousands of different invoice, purchase order, and bill of lading documents! Despite widespread acceptance of standard code sets and standard paper claim forms, claim processing procedures are not uniform across the country. Different payers request different data content even though a standard paper form is used. Many payers request attachments of other reports, such as the emergency room report or the operating room report, before paying a claim. In addition, many managed care contracts include reimbursement calculations that are impossible to bill on the standard claim form. The value of EDI format standards is severely compromised if industry participants do not have a commitment to uniform data content standards.

In the healthcare industry during the 1980s, all of the movement to X12 standards took place in material management applications. The Health Industry Bar Coding Council, which was once only concerned with bar code standards, evolved to become the Healthcare Information Business Communications Council (HIBCC). HIBCC's membership consists of distributors, manufacturers, and providers. Its expanded charter deals with healthcare applications of X12 EDI standards such as purchase orders, shipping notices, and invoices. HIBCC publishes implementation manuals that contain the X12 standards with advice on how they should be implemented by healthcare providers and their vendors. Healthcare EDI for material management applications appears to be following the pattern of other industries. Manufacturers that supported proprietary communications systems for purchase orders and related transactions from providers are moving to use the X12 standards.

A more recent catalyst for widespread adoption of EDI in the healthcare industry is its adoption by those who fund and administer provider reimbursement. As important as the purchase process is for most providers, its automation through EDI can provide only a fraction of the benefits available from a comparable automation of the information exchanged between payers and providers.

Although the insurance industry overall has many traditions of developing standards, it was a latecomer to the ANSI process. The first discussions about ANSI ASC X12 standards for insurance began in 1989. Since then the standards development work in the Insurance Subcommittee of the X12 organization (X12N) has moved quickly. In the healthcare arena, the rapid pace of standards development can be attributed to a consensus shared among both the claims payers and healthcare providers that the administrative costs of health care can be substantially lowered by using EDI.

The case for the efficiency of electronic claims submission has been proven by the Medicare program, in which the Health Care Financing Administration (HCFA) receives the overwhelming majority of its Part A claims from hospitals electronically. The federal government is an active proponent of electronic commerce and its Federal Information Processing Standard (FIPS) requires federal agencies to use ANSI X12 standards for electronic data interchange when an appropriate standard is available. Since 1991, HCFA has been working closely with providers, private sector payers, and other members of the X12 standards development group. HCFA's stated goal of being paperless by the year 2000 will be met through the use of X12 EDI.

OTHER STANDARDS

Several important organizations in addition to ANSI have been involved in developing standards for health care. Medical records professionals who have the responsibility for the patient records have a great interest in computer-based patient records. Medical records professionals have a national association known as the

AHIMA, the American Health Information Management Association. These professionals will play an important role in the electronic exchange of clinical data, but the data that goes into the electronic patient record is now standardized by a host of specialized organizations. The radiology industry has developed standards for the digital imaging of x-rays, and the sponsoring organizations are the American College of Radiology and the National Electronic Manufacturers Association (ACR-NEMA). Their radiology standard is known as DICOM 3. A laboratory standards was developed by the American Society for Testing and Materials (ASTM). A widely used standard for the transmission of real-time pharmacy claims was developed by the National Council for Prescription Drug Programs (NCPDP).

The development of many different electronic standards by different players in the healthcare industry bears a striking resemblance to comparable developments in industry-specific standards. Standards were first devised for narrow solutions and subsequent attempts at standardization were attempted for industry-wide solutions. Today many of these organizations are working to harmonize their standardization efforts. The history of lab reporting standards provides a good example. The two organizations involved are ASTM and Health Level 7 (HL7).

ASTM is a nonprofit organization founded in 1898. It has become one of the largest voluntary standards development systems in the world. In 1970, ASTM organized the Committee on Computerized Laboratory Systems (Committee E-31) to prepare standards for parts of the system development process such as definition, implementation, documentation, and evaluation. In 1991 ASTM Specification E1238 was initially developed for clinical laboratory results. ASTM revised Standard E1238 and it is now referred to as Specification E 1238-91 . In this revision, the scope has been extended to most kinds of clinical data, including physicians' and nurses' notes, imaging results, and more.

HL7 is an organization whose scope includes all information exchanges among the information application programs within a hospital. Many hospitals and their system vendors support HL7 standards. The need for HL7 grew out of the challenge of linking a pharmacy system made by one vendor to the material management system of another and the patient accounting system of a

FIGURE 2–1

HL7 standards were developed to connect different clinical and adminis-
trative software used in a medical setting. This figure shows some of the
programs that may be connected on a local area network using HL7
standards in a hospital setting.

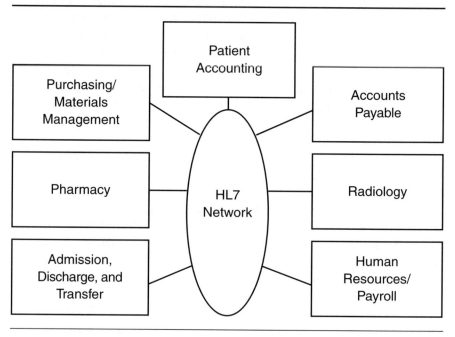

third vendor. Figure 2–1 illustrates the variety of systems in a hospital that may exchange data through the use of HL7 standards.
Many laboratory reports do not involve hospitals as trading partners, but the HL7 and ASTM standards developers coordinated
development so the standards are quite similar.

HL7 developers have also been working with X12 standards
developers. The HL7 standards are designed for use within a hospital and not for transmission among different organizations—that
is the task of X12 EDI standards. In fact a representative of the HL7
organization, Community Medical Center of Scranton, Pennsylva-
nia, placed the request with ASC X12 to develop a claim standard.

The difference may be somewhat confusing at first. A comparison with the way we do business in a paper-based world may be

helpful. Data conforming to HL7 standards can be sent between hospital systems in a fashion similar to an interoffice memo. By contrast, a letter is put into the mail and sent to another organization and this requires support of specific mail standards. First of all, a standard-sized envelope must be used, then receiver and sender address information must be placed in standardized locations on the envelope. X12 EDI standards provide the envelope and transmission format for interorganizational transmission. Standard developers within X12 do not wish to support data element definitions that are specific to a particular industry. They look to industry organizations to support those needs. For example, the data elements on the National Uniform Bill, the UB 92, are incorporated by reference into the X12 claim standard, the Health Care Claim (837). This differentiation between data content standards (for example, industry agreement about how laboratory test values should be expressed or codes used for claims submission) and format standards (EDI X12 formats) should be clear.

The fully networked healthcare community will require that this information be exchanged among participants in the industry. In recognition of that need, the Healthcare Informatics Standards Planning Panel was created under ANSI auspices for the groups to coordinate standardization efforts to avoid duplication.

The standards that govern the transmission of data also need to be discussed. E-mail, in particular, is an important tool that compliments EDI.

EDI AND ELECTRONIC MAIL

How does the use of electronic mail (E-mail) relate to EDI? Many organizations have used E-mail for internal communications since the 1980s. Organizations may use an E-mail system called PROFS if they have IBM computers or VMS Mail if they have Digital Equipment (DEC) computers. Many PC users now use E-mail within a local area network. How do E-mail and EDI differ?

By definition, EDI is used for computer-to-computer transmissions without any human intervention. E-mail is meant to be read by the person addressed. Although EDI transactions can contain text messages, the practice is frowned upon because the business mission of EDI is data exchange without any human intervention and its related costs. Another difference between the two is that most E-mail users are exchanging the electronic equivalent of interoffice memos with coworkers. They seldom exchange E-mail messages with people outside their organizations. In contrast, most EDI exchanges are among different companies.

Despite discouraging text messages, EDI advocates recognize the business need for electronic messaging between different organizations. Any avid user of EDI within an organization has undoubtedly wished to send messages to outsiders. Unfortunately, the E-mail capability of most companies usually does not extend beyond their walls. Why can't E-mail messages be sent to people in other organizations? The problem again is lack of standards: The E-mail system of one organization may not "talk" to the system of the other. In other words, E-mail is used mainly with propriety standards (as was originally the case with EDI). National or international standards are needed to send text messages electronically.

In 1984, an international communications standards body introduced an international standard for E-mail or "interpersonal messaging" (to use the phrasing of the standard).[3] This standard was designated X.400 because it was introduced as Recommendation Number 400.[4] It is still the most widely supported version of the standard, although other versions were released in 1988 and 1990. Because both intercorporate EDI and E-mail have been growing it is appropriate that the 1990 version of X.400 has been extended to include a new EDI-specific protocol called X.435. This new standard allows a sender to put together electronic data of different types into one package for one receiver. In the corporate world that might include an X12 purchase order (850), an electronic blueprint file (a computer-aided design/computer-aided manufacturing file or CAD/CAM file), and a fax message. In the provider community, a patient accounting department could send an X12

---

[3] *EDI News*, August 10, 1992.

[4] There has been some confusion about the pronunciation of X.400 as providers are simultaneously learning about X12 standards. The use of the designation "X" in both is coincidental, because these standards have been developed by different organizations. The word *dot* is not used in the pronunciation of X.400.

claim transaction (837) and a fax of the operative report to a payer. A hospital could also send demographic data about a patient to a nursing home in an X12 format that could be captured by the patient accounting system of the nursing home and also include a text message comprising a hospital discharge summary.

The X.400 standard is reportedly more widely used internationally than in the United States. The U.S. aerospace industry moved to the widespread use of X.400 years ago because the trading partners in the industry saw it as a necessity. So have many participants in the defense industry. Imagine the needs of a defense contractor dealing with subcontractors all over the country. With the leadership of the U.S. Department of Defense, EDI and E-mail have been supported in that industry as well. E-mail has a tremendous role in linking all the participants in the healthcare industry as well.

The long-term cost of creating electronic linkages in health care will depend on the development and support of standards through the organizations described in this chapter. The healthcare industry needs to fund and support the development of additional EDI standards to completely automate their interactions with important trading partners. The challenge for the industry is to educate leadership and management about the role of standards and the importance of uniform implementation. The debate about healthcare reform initiated by the Clinton Administration illustrated the extensive disapproval, shared by all participants, of the exorbitant costs of paperwork in the administration of health care. The healthcare industry can either work through the challenge of standardization by itself or be condemned for wastefulness and risk government intervention to cure the problem.

Chapter Three

Electronic Networks

For many managers in the healthcare industry a network consists of a group of contracted providers. This chapter deals with different kinds of networks that can be used to exchange information among different organizations in the industry.

The information systems (IS) professionals in most organizations have spent the bulk of their time supporting software and the computers on which it runs. In the past, information could be moved from one computer to another through the exchange of tapes. More recently, many organizations have installed local area networks (LANs) through which computers exchange information using cables strung among them. The challenge of moving information by telecommunications is often a new experience to IS professionals and business managers, and the insights of experienced EDI users is valuable. A key component to the successful implementation of EDI in corporate America is the role of the value added network (VAN).

THE ROLE OF THE VAN

LANs enable computers to be connected by dedicated cables on the same floor or in the same building. How are computers that are in different buildings, different cities, and perhaps different states to be connected when cables cannot be used? The answer has been to use the telephone lines that already connect companies. Digital data is regularly transmitted over phone lines using modems. Some larger organizations have telecommunications departments and an array of modems for different types of data transfers.

Phones and modems will be the prime mechanisms to facilitate electronic networks in health care, but additional services are needed. As other industries turned to phones and modems to handle EDI, they discovered that there was a complex management task in tracking all the connections. The first challenge faced was one of time. Different companies wanted to do their EDI exchanges at different times and not remain ready to send and receive messages all day. Many healthcare claims payers, for example, might dedicate their systems to an end-of-week or end-of-month process, so the necessary programs would not be available to electronically respond to a provider's eligibility inquiry.

Another complication that arose was one of technical compatibilities among different modem protocols and different line speeds. Electronic trading partners realized that although business should be done by phone, some service provider was needed to manage the equivalent of an electronic postal service. VANs provide such services and have played a major role in the expansion of EDI.

VAN services are provided by many major corporations including General Electric, AT&T, and IBM, among others. Business managers who are new to networks should think of VANS as essentially large computers with many phone connections. The principal service VANs offer is called a *store-and-forward service.* It is an electronic counterpart to the postal service. Rather than deliver mail directly to all recipients, correspondents submit mail to the postal service, which in turn delivers mail to the receivers. VANs offer a comparable service and store messages received to be forwarded to recipient trading partners. This enables the sender to be responsible for maintaining only one telecommunications connection rather than many. This also eliminates the need to schedule transmissions to meet the needs of the receiving party.

VANs are used by many companies in many industries, including health care. Many hospitals use VANs to transmit electronic purchase orders and confirmations. Some claims payers also use VANs to collect electronic claims and transmit remittance information to providers. In addition, services comparable to those of VANs have been provided by organizations called claims clearing-houses. These companies provide reformatting services and deliver claims gathered from many providers to payers. Clearing-houses developed in part because of the lack of an EDI standard for claims and they helped providers cope with different payer requirements for electronic billing.

In addition to electronic claim traffic transmitted in a store-and-forward process, the pharmacy industry processes claims in a "real time" or interactive mode. Pharmacy claims are simpler and contain less data than medical claims and are well suited for inter-active processing. Interactive processing is a network service that is more akin to the communications linkages that connect auto-matic teller machines (ATMs) and credit card processors. Many companies that have the capability to provide real time message transport see a bright future for "interactive EDI," particularly for eligibility transactions. Interactive processing is not appropriate for larger electronic exchanges such as clinical information between providers or large enrollment files sent from an employer to a benefits administrator.

THE ELECTRONIC MAILROOM

Although many vendors and journalists are describing the task of "building healthcare networks," readers should not be misled into thinking that vast amounts of fiber optic cables need to be laid to complete the task. As just described, phone lines already in place can readily handle the load now transmitted on paper through the mail in an EDI system. What is not in place for the networking of health care is the electronic mailroom, a combination of software and hardware linkages to the network and business practices for doing business electronically.

In corporate America the approach to EDI has often been to acquire EDI software and to create an *EDI team* to implement con-nections with trading partners. (Chapter 9, "Organizing for EDI," describes the structure and role of the EDI team.) The EDI team is responsible for obtaining downloaded information from internal application programs when the information is destined for out-bound transactions. The EDI team also is responsible for receiving incoming EDI messages and creating the proper upload file for processing in the organization's internal application program. Corporate trading partners often engage in a bilateral exchange of trading partner agreements that cover legal issues related to paperless purchasing and payments. Major hospital systems may use the same business approach with their EDI links to suppliers.

EDI for claim traffic dwarfs all procurement-related EDI, and the business model for claim processing is quite different from practices in corporate America. Hospital providers often use claim clearinghouses that provide a service of obtaining downloaded claims from patient accounting programs and subsequently rout-ing the claims to payers. Doctors' offices produce far more claims than do hospitals, and hundreds of vendors of claims clearing-house services transmit claims for physicians. Many vendors of patient accounting systems or physician practice management sys-tems also provide electronic claims services. Providers that rely on claim clearinghouse services have outsourced part of the manage-ment of their electronic mailroom. Providers that want to support their own communications with trading partners will probably acquire EDI software to assist in the task.

SOFTWARE FOR USE OF THE NETWORK

Software tools have been developed to make the use of standard EDI formats much easier. Organizations that want to exchange data need not change their internal programs or the formats they wish to use to send or receive data. The EDI standard format is used to convey information among organizations with different hardware and software configurations. A familiar analogy for this process is the way in which information is exchanged at the United Nations. Most nations send translators who are familiar with the country's native language and with English, the standard language used for communication. Each country's translator is capable of translating from English back into the native language, and vice versa. Several countries—none of whom has English as a native language—can all exchange information through the standard communication language.

In a comparable fashion EDI trading partners translate data from internal formats used by their application programs into and out of the standard EDI format. As might be expected, EDI software is often called a *translator* because it reformats a file from the originating computer into the EDI standard and translates from the EDI standard to the receiving computer's format. EDI software can enable any computer hardware and software configuration to communicate with any other. Hardware and software "compatibility" is not required among trading partners. EDI software can be used in a mainframe, minicomputer, or personal computer regardless of proprietary operating systems or hardware architectures at either end. Larger companies may choose mainframe or minicomputer EDI software, but most EDI software is PC-based. Software for larger computers may be more expensive, but PC-based EDI software has become readily available and inexpensive. Limited-function packages are available for less than $1,000 and more loaded packages cost less than $4,000.

This software may combine translation functions with communications capabilities. The communications software is similar to file transfer programs used whenever a computer is connected via a modem to communications services.

In addition to communications and translation functionalities, two other functions may be part of an EDI management software package: mapping and interchange control.

The *mapping function* automates a process that can be done on paper by determining where a piece of data in one file format should be placed in another format. This can be time consuming and EDI users that will be supporting many EDI exchanges might find mapping functionality a helpful component in the EDI package the organization selects.

Interchange control is an important aspect of EDI software. Interchange control enables trading partners to manage message traffic. For example, exchanges between trading partners are numbered sequentially, so that if a claim payer was sent claims number 1,256 and 1,257 from a provider and the prior transactions were numbered 1,243 and 1,244, the payer could notify the provider that the intervening numbered transactions had not been received.

ELECTRONIC COMMERCE AND COMMUNITY HEALTHCARE INFORMATION NETWORKS

Corporate America is now adopting the phrase *electronic commerce* to encompass EDI, E-mail, electronic forms, and other paperless exchanges. Magazines and organizations founded to deal with EDI are changing their names and the scope of their interests to include the non-EDI aspects of electronic commerce. Somehow that name does not fit the healthcare industry. With its primary focus on patient care and the tax-exempt, community health improvement nature of the mission of many of its institutions, the phrase *electronic commerce* seems inappropriate for health care. Providers will adopt the tools of electronic commerce but for their own unique purposes and with their own vocabulary.

Rather than saying they participate in electronic commerce, providers may participate in a *community healthcare information network (CHIN).* The vision of moving both clinical and administrative information electronically throughout the healthcare community was first widely discussed through the efforts of the John A. Hartford Foundation. That charitable trust funded master plans to illustrate how community networks might work and provided "seed capital" in the form of grants to interested communities. The first three grants provided by the Hartford Foundation went to sponsors in the states of Washington and Iowa and the city of Memphis, Tennessee, in 1992. The goal of a CHIN is to link all the trading partners involved in health care in an effort to reduce costs and practice better medicine.

Although the definition of a CHIN is simple, there are differing approaches for setting up a CHIN. Some proponents envision the CHIN as having a central data repository—a central mainframe computer where data collected from all community participants is warehoused. However, many difficult sociopolitical issues surround the concept of a central repository: Who owns the data, who maintains it, who has access to it, and how big can the database be? An alternative format allows the CHIN to be developed by a sponsor (an HMO, a healthcare system, or a business coalition) that can access all the information available while enabling each facility to own and maintain its own database. The CHIN manager in this alternative approach acts more like a librarian with procedures for tapping into many electronic libraries rather than a custodian of one master database.

In some states, such as Iowa, all payers and providers will be required by legislation to participate in a CHIN. In other areas participation is voluntary. Other market forces are propelling the healthcare industry into more extensive networking, particularly the movement to managed care.

MANAGED CARE AS A CATALYST FOR HEALTHCARE NETWORKS

HCFA played a key role in forcing the adoption of standards for claims-related EDI. Managed care will play a comparable role in accelerating provider-to-provider EDI. (See Chapter 5 for a description of EDI uses in managed care.)

There are two reasons for this:

- *Managed care practices are time-sensitive and transaction intensive.* Managed care certification has shifted the attention of the hospital patient accounting department from linking with payers to linking with physicians. The hospital has to link electronically with the medical groups, independent practitioner associations (IPAs), and HMOs that certify care. If certification is not managed and tracked the hospital will not get paid. This administrative requirement of managed care will motivate provider-to-provider EDI linkages.

- *Managed care organizations will have to measure outcomes in ways that will require information collection in electronic patient records by the provider community.* Providers and HMOs will have to prove to employers and other plan sponsors that they meet the standards now being developed for "managed care report cards." One example of such reporting requirements is the HEDIS data set supported by many of the larger managed care organizations and employer coalitions. Other business coalitions have developed other, more extensive, measurements to ensure that managed care companies compete on both the cost and the quality of care.

In contrast to a CHIN, initiatives for networking health systems that seek to network physicians and hospitals to compete more effectively in a managed care environment are referred to as *enterprise model CHINs* or simply as *health information networks (HINs)*.

HOW PHYSICIAN-HOSPITAL NETWORKING CAN BE MANAGED

The new dimension added by either the CHIN or HIN will be provider-to-provider EDI with an explicit commitment from participants to move toward a transmittable electronic patient record. Electronic exchanges between providers will be both clinical and administrative in nature. Is this totally new? Not really. Hospital laboratories may already be doing electronic reporting of results to physicians, most often by fax or by using remote terminals. The shift in emphasis will be that such exchanges should become standard operating procedure. Software now displayed in physician's office vendor shows illustrates the new focus on electronic clinical data. The latest software for physicians can receive HL7 and ASTM standard electronic reports from local hospitals. Clinical patient record capabilities are now accompanying traditional invoice generation and patient scheduling modules for the physician's office. Physicians and hospitals have always worked together, and now electronic connections will play a greater role in their relationship, reinforced by joint contracting with managed care organizations.

A larger issue is how hospitals will organize and manage the overall electronic relationship between physician and hospital. Will three departments within a hospital concoct three different ways of connecting to physicians electronically, rather than present one solution that works for all three departments? Will hospitals have a conscious strategy of building relationships with physicians with the tools used in corporate America in electronic commerce?

The technology is available and the standards are available, but today these tasks are not part of anyone's job description at most provider organizations. For all the technical network wizardry available today, successful providers will have to adopt a conscious network strategy and intelligently manage the conversion from paper to electronic processing.

II

HEALTHCARE APPLICATIONS FOR EDI

Chapter Four

EDI for the Claim Process

This chapter explores in depth the differences between paper-based and electronic claims processing and notes the benefits of implementing EDI to streamline the claims process.

THE PRICE OF NONSTANDARD PROCESSING

Healthcare providers are continually criticized for the capital they have tied up in unoccupied beds and in underused, high-technology equipment. Yet during the 1980s hospitals invested billions of

FIGURE 4–1
Patient accounting timeline for claims.

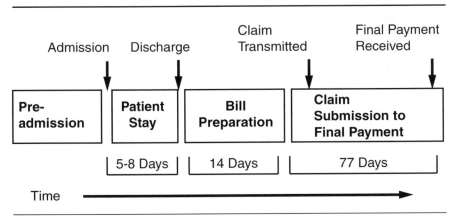

dollars in higher levels of accounts receivable. This is as wasteful as building facilities to sit unoccupied in the desert. The waste inherent in this unproductive use of capital is matched by theenormous expense of feeding the paper mill known as the administration of health care. In early 1991 an article in the *New England Journal of Medicine* compared the administrative costs of the U.S. healthcare system with Canadian levels.[1] The authors of the article calculated that just under 25 percent of every healthcare dollar was spend on administrative overhead. The comparable Canadian figures were 8 to 11 percent. A quick calculation showed that if U.S. health care were as administratively efficient as the Canadian system, Americans could save nearly $81 billion—enough to provide insurance for every uninsured American. This comparison set off a firestorm of criticism. Such coverage was combined with the November 1991 senatorial race in Pennsylvania that revolved around a "healthcare reform" platform. This debate served as a catalyst in bringing many participants into the ANSI X12 EDI process to create national electronic standards for healthcare insurance transactions.

Today's paper-based procedures for provider payments not only create a huge working capital requirement but are also a significant provider operating expense. Billing and collection functions within a hospital are a major component of total hospital administrative costs. A 500-bed hospital may require as many as 100 patient accounting employees to keep up with the paperwork load. In parts of the country where managed care companies have a significant presence, the reporting requirements before and during the provision of services have required additional employees to handle the workload. Table 4–1 illustrates the relative cost of the patient accounting function as a percentage of total hospital administrative and fiscal expenses.

The table's numbers illustrate the substantial expense related to patient billing. Clearly, if the process could be automated these

---

[1] See Steffie Woolhandler and David U. Himmelstein, "The Deteriorating Administrative Efficiency and the U.S. Health Care System," *New England Journal of Medicine* 324: 1253-58 (May 2, 1991) and Robert G. Evans et al., "Controlling Health Expenditures: The Canadian Reality," *New England Journal of Medicine* 320: 571-577 (March 2, 1989). See also the journal's three-part series on the Canadian healthcare system published in 1986 in volumes 315 and 316.

TABLE 4–1
Median Hospital Administrative and Fiscal Expenses—January to June 1992

Hospital bed size	100–149	150–199	200–299	300–399	400+
	Direct expense per adjusted occupied bed				
Total administrative/ fiscal	$2220	$2222	$2246	$2436	$2614
Administration	1090	1072	1088	1065	1078
Patient accounts/ admitting	520	521	448	440	456
General accounting	177	162	139	134	120
Data processing	254	220	235	283	391
	Percentage of total administrative and fiscal expenses				
Administration	47.65	48.54	50.03	48.24	43.94
Patient accounts/ admitting	22.97	22.71	20.16	18.32	18.56
General accounting	7.63	6.61	5.88	4.86	4.69
Data processing	9.77	9.81	10.66	11.70	13.50

Source: American Hospital Association, *Monitrend II.* Copyright AHA, 1992.

expenses could be significantly reduced. Automation has not occurred for two major reasons:

- There have been no standards until recently for the electronic exchange of the relevant information.
- There has been declining industry consensus about what information should be exchanged between payer and provider.

We pay a high price as a society for not putting our house in order. Some providers and claims payers have lapsed into a permanent adversarial attitude toward their trading partners. Benefit administrators and providers must come to an agreement about how they are going to do business. The development and use of EDI standards will be a consensus-creating process of crucial importance for the industry.

Why is the claims process so difficult for the average provider? The healthcare claim itself is a complex combination of clinical and billing data elements that have been somewhat standardized in a paper format. The claim is not just an invoice for medical services. It performs a variety of functions for different constituencies because it is an important means of gathering healthcare data as well as billing for it.

Physicians' services are usually billed on a form called the HCFA 1500, which is approved by the Health Care Financing Administration (HCFA) for services rendered under Medicare Part B coverage. (Medicare offers Part A coverage for hospital inpatient services and Part B coverage for outpatient services.) The UB 92 (Uniform Bill 1992 revision) was developed by the National Uniform Billing Committee, which has payer and provider representation and is sponsored by the American Hospital Association. This form is used as a summary bill for hospital inpatient services and is accepted by most payers. In recent years its usefulness has been compromised by the many payers that ask for additional information before processing payment.

The claim process is difficult for providers because healthcare insurance in the United States is provided by myriad organizations and a patchwork of programs. Calls for single-payer systems or "payment reform" highlight the confusing nature of how we pay for health care. The claims process does not make sense without an understanding of who pays for health care. It is worth a short review to identify the players and to clear up some common misunderstandings about payment delays.

HEALTHCARE TRADING PARTNERS: WHO PAYS THE BILLS?

Most Americans have some level of healthcare insurance provided for them by their employers as part of an employee benefit program. Since 1964, the federal government's Medicare program has provided insurance for the elderly. Simultaneously, Medicaid was begun as the state and federally funded program to provide means-tested health insurance coverage. These three funding sources (employers, Medicare, and Medicaid) pay for about 90 percent of the nation's annual healthcare spending. Individuals may buy healthcare insurance directly and frequently also contribute a portion of the cost of employer-provided insurance through payroll deductions. Because healthcare insurance frequently requires the beneficiary to absorb a portion of the cost of treatment, the total cost of health care for individuals comes from both insurance costs and out-of-pocket expenses.

Additional complexity arises in the system because payments are made under different reimbursement methodologies. In the past, claims were paid based on provider charges, but fee schedule schemes determined by different payers have proliferated. These schemes include the Medicare Prospective Payment System and contractual reimbursement arrangements for managed care and preferred provider organizations. Dealing with all of these variations is anything but simple. The patient accounting staff spend a great deal of time on the phone obtaining eligibility information, dealing with the utilization review process, and inquiring about the status of claims and expected payments.

The Use of Float

Because the payment process takes so much time, many providers feel that claims payers are using the opportunity to make significant investment income on "float" or undisbursed funds. Investment income can be earned by insurance companies on funds that are received as premium income before those funds are disbursed for claims payments and administrative expenses. The longer the period between collection and disbursement, the greater the income from investments. This view of how payers conduct their business is at the root of the ill will some providers have toward the payer community. In fact, the trend toward self-insurance among corporate employers (including many hospitals) has led to a situation in which most claim payers do not insure their customers but only process the claims for an administrative fee. Because they are not paid premiums, the companies that administer healthcare benefit programs do not have the funds available for investment. In many cases, insurance companies no longer insure against risk; their function is to administer reimbursement. This development merits detailed explanation because suspicions about payer motivations can distort the payer/provider dialog.

In the past, most employers and individuals paid premiums to insurance companies that spread the risk of loss over a large base of customers. Blue Cross Blue Shield plans provided insurance that was "community rated," that is, the loss experience of an entire region or community determined the premium for those who applied for insurance. Commercial insurance companies grew by offering group insurance to large employers based on the loss experience of that large group of employees. Both of these traditional insurance products have lost ground in recent years to self-insurance programs.

ASOs and TPAs

Self-insured organizations that provide healthcare benefits for their employees or members do not pay premiums to an insurance company. Actuaries are retained to estimate probable losses, and the appropriate level of funding is made to a trust account. Insurance companies, acting as *administrative service only (ASO) processors* for the benefit plan, or independent companies known as *third-party administrators (TPAs)* are then hired to process claims for a fee frequently priced on a charge per claim. The checks printed for claims payments are drawn on the trust account for the benefit plan, not on funds whose investment income accrues to the administrator or claims processor. Those who accuse claim payers of delaying claim payments to benefit from the float are incorrect. The claim processor has every incentive to lower administrative costs and streamline the process.

New Model for Information Flow among Trading Partners

These new business relationships have been incorporated into the terminology in the ANSI X12 standards. A model for the major trading partner relationships is emerging as the standards process progresses. In the model the plan sponsor is the ultimate buyer of

FIGURE 4–2
Principal healthcare claim information flows.

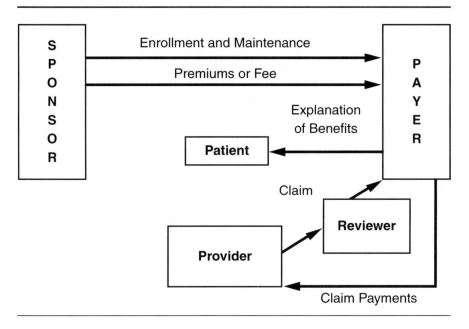

healthcare insurance. Plan sponsors can be employers, government agencies, and individuals who select the terms and conditions of insurance coverage and the benefits available. Healthcare providers are those who provide medical services for patients who receive care. Reimbursement for services rendered by providers is made by payers who administer the insurance benefits purchased by sponsors. Finally, reviewers such as utilization review firms or preferred provider organizations may be contracted by the payer or the plan sponsor to examine treatment plans or the pricing of medical services. Figure 4–2 diagrams some of the principal information flows between sponsors, payers, reviewers, providers, and patients.

Premium or administrative billing and payment may be accommodated by existing EDI standards, but a new standard was needed for the repetitive transactions that deal with enrollment. Sponsors continually send demographic data to payers to maintain the accuracy of a list of covered individuals. The list is subject to changes from births, marriages, deaths, retirements, and employee turnover. Covered individuals may also select different benefits, levels of deductibles, and other variables, and these benefit selections must be transmitted to the payer. The accuracy of the payer's enrollment file is important to all trading partners. It controls the premium and administrative fee determination for the sponsor and is used by the provider (in non-life-threatening situations) to assess the patient's ability to pay the costs associated with care.

One of the first EDI standards for healthcare insurance deals with this information flow. It began life as "Healthcare Enrollment and Maintenance," but its designers soon realized that the sponsor-to-payer information flow dealt with a larger array of benefits. Healthcare benefits are only a portion of an overall employee benefits program for the corporate employer. The standard now allows for the transmission of information about disability insurance, life insurance, retirement savings, and flexible-spending accounts. It has been appropriately renamed "Benefit Enrollment and Maintenance." The Benefit Enrollment and Maintenance (834) standard can be used for the transmission of all demographic information when a sponsor selects a new payer, and it can be used for ongoing additions, changes, and deletions to an existing payer enrollment file.

Sponsors, payers, and providers will all benefit from the widespread adoption of the 834 and the elimination of inaccurate or untimely transfer of enrollment information. Sponsors who are tardy or inaccurate in transmitting this information suffer in a variety of ways. Benefits may be paid for ineligible patients who would have been removed from the enrollment file if information were passed in a timely manner. Premium or administrative fee payments may be inaccurate when payers and sponsors find that their enrollment lists do not correspond. When the payer's enrollment list is out-of-date, providers suffer losses because they provide care for patients who are ineligible and who cannot pay the bill from their personal resources. The information exchange during enrollment must be accurate, or the information will corrupt the business efficiency of every transaction that follows. (See Chapter 7, "EDI for the Human Resource Department," for additional information on the use of the 834.)

THE CLAIMS PROCESS UNDER EDI

Many healthcare providers think of the claims process in terms of the administration of the patient accounting process within their own organizations. Jobs are designed and work distributed internally to ensure rapid collection of physicians' discharge summaries, fast turnaround by medical coders, and diligent collection efforts on unpaid claims. Similarly, payers develop flow charts that track the information flows within their organization. Both payers and providers apply many different techniques to reduce errors and speed up the work flow. The development of EDI standards for provider and payer information exchanges redefines the work flow to focus on the information exchanged between payer and provider in addition to information gathered and processed internally. Figure 4–3 summarizes the claim process and the major exchanges between payer and provider.

FIGURE 4–3
EDI standard transactions for the claims process.

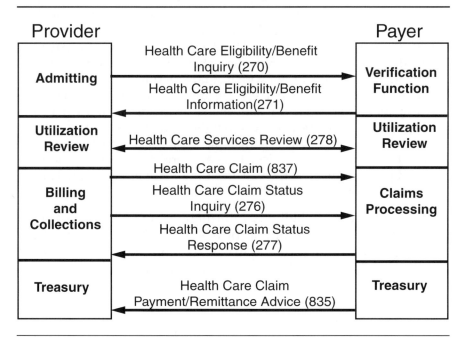

Eligibility Inquiry and Response

Eligibility inquiry is the first exchange between payer and provider in the claims process. Most patient accounting professionals concur that the speed with which claims will be paid does not just depend on the actions taken after a claim is submitted but by actions taken earlier in the timeline—particularly before medical treatment is provided. For inpatient hospital admissions, the key point for applying EDI is the preadmission process, because the quality of information obtained during this phase is crucial to the successful collection of payment.

Mary Bednar, assistant director of finance at the University of Virginia Medical Center (UVAMC), takes advantage of a variety of electronic applications to improve efficiency. She states that:

> Through Health Communication Services (HCS), a wholly owned subsidiary of Blue Cross Blue Shield of Virginia, UVAMC is able to check the eligibility status of patients against the Medicare Common Working File, the State of Virginia Medicaid list of eligible recipients, and the enrolled subscribers of Blue Cross Blue Shield of Virginia. UVAMC can confirm whether the insurance coverage claimed by a patient is current or has lapsed. In addition, the benefit details of different Blue Cross Blue Shield contracts can be obtained and reviewed in depth with the patient. This enables UVAMC to collect correct copayment and deductible amounts from the patient before discharge. Patients may not be fully conversant with insurance terminology and coverage details. UVAMC staff members can discuss payment arrangements with patients and explain what benefits are available and what costs must be borne by the patient or another payer. Electronic eligibility and benefit inquiry ensures that the basic demographic data and expected reimbursement calculations are correct. In addition, the automated process enhances the patient's confidence in the hospital and is a valuable customer service.[2]

The availability of eligibility information from all payers will be aided by widespread adoption of ANSI standards known as the Health Benefit Eligibility Inquiry (270) and the Health Benefit Eligibility Information (271). The problem of eligibility is more

---

[2] James J. Moynihan and Kathryn C. Norman, "Claims Submission Leads Electronic Advances," *Healthcare Financial Management* (June 1992), pp. 83-84.

complex than it might appear, and a number of attempts to supply eligibility information to providers have been unsuccessful, in part because there are different definitions of what constitutes eligibility. Providers lump different questions into eligibility. They tend to combine two questions: "Is this person enrolled in a benefit plan and thus eligible for reimbursement?" and "Is this service a covered benefit?" Providers want to know, of course, whether the services they provide will be paid for. They desire instant adjudication, which is reasonable for all types of organizations that want to minimize credit losses.

Unfortunately, it is getting harder to answer these questions. As described by Mary Bednar, UVAMC is able to determine copayment and deductible amounts based on a plan whose conditions apply to many individuals. The trend in employee benefits is to provide greater choice for the employee and greater customization of benefits. Rather than using a single plan for all members in a community or all employees of a given employer, individuals can use "cafeteria style" benefit plans to customize the priorities among their benefits. Flexible spending arrangements add to the customization options, as do point-of-service plans. These plans enable employees to choose the reimbursement procedure at the time medical service is rendered. Point-of-service choices include indemnity coverage that allows complete freedom to choose a provider with limited reimbursement; a preferred provider option that limits providers but increases coverage; and an exclusive provider option that sharply curtails freedom of choice for the employee but offers the most generous coverage. Although such a broad range of benefit plans may be an attractive employment incentive for the sponsor's human resource department, the plans create an administrative nightmare for the provider.

This complexity illustrates the point that the accuracy of the data used in the claims process is determined by what takes place between sponsor and payer. The benefit plan design has a large impact on the ability of the provider to estimate reimbursement. In addition to the accuracy of the enrollee list and the terms of coverage details, the scope of services eligible for reimbursement is a factor.

All too often plan documents are written in legal terms that are subject to varying interpretation by different claim examiners. Benefit coverage codes are developed by payers to cover certain procedure and diagnosis codes submitted by providers. Different payers using the same plan document might develop different benefit codes. This is becoming more apparent to standards designers working on the response to an eligibility inquiry. The industry needs a set of standard benefit codes for all payers. These codes will affect the way in which sponsors develop plan documents at the beginning of the claim process. Discovering this interrelationship of plan documents and process codes is indicative of how working to develop an EDI solution reveals ways to improve the entire process.

Claims Submission

Healthcare claims are the principle documents exchanged between payers and providers. The transaction volumes are enormous: Some 5 billion claims are filed each year in the United States. Less than 20 percent of these claims were exchanged electronically in 1995; the rest were paper forms and supporting documentation. Despite this low overall percentage, electronic claims submission is frequently used by hospitals to submit Medicare claims. The overwhelming majority of America's hospitals submit Medicare Part A (inpatient) claims electronically. Electronic claims submission is changing rapidly as new technologies are used.

Electronic claim submission in one form or another has been in use for 20 years. The earliest applications sprang up as payers and providers exchanged magnetic tapes containing claims data rather than mailing paper claims forms. In addition to the exchange of tapes, Blue Cross organizations often placed "dumb" computer terminals in the business offices of major providers. Direct telephone lines (leased lines) connected these terminals to the mainframe computer of the Blue Cross plan. During the 1970s HCFA provided incentives to fiscal intermediaries in the Medicare program to promote such leased line linkages. Providers were encouraged to use direct data entry (DDE) terminals to key claims data directly into the claims adjudication system of the fiscal intermediary. This resulted in faster payment, because claims no longer spent time in the mail or in a pile of paper awaiting data entry. HCFA and its intermediaries benefited, because the cost of data entry was shifted to the provider.

DDE remained the most prevalent form of electronic claim submission in the 1980s. Technological advances and changing business practices should eliminate DDE in the 1990s, however. Electronic claim submission software has been selected by many providers to replace direct data entry terminals. Although such programs can be installed on a hospital mainframe or a minicomputer, most are used on PCs as claims editor workstations. As PC prices decreased and their computing power increased, the attractiveness of a networked PC installation has increased.

In a typical installation, the PC is configured to receive claims that are electronically "downloaded" from the patient accounting system. Claims thus received are then edited and telecommunicated either directly to a payer or through a claims submission vendor to the payer. This procedure offers several important advantages over prior DDE methods. DDE required data to be rekeyed from a printed patient bill. The elimination of repetitive data entry tasks speeds claims submission while decreasing staffing required. In addition, claim edits can help managers to generate more "clean claims"—ones without errors. These advantages result in faster payment of claims at lower costs.

Providers expect electronic claims submission to result in faster claims payments. Ken Morgan, patient accounting manager at Wheeling Hospital in Wheeling, West Virginia, has witnessed the transition from direct data entry for claims to the use of a PC claim submission program in two hospitals. According to Ken, "Both hospitals experienced a reduction in their outstanding days in accounts receivable." At Wheeling Hospital, a 276-bed facility with 14,000 admissions and 114,000 outpatient visits a year, the transition took place in early 1991. "Within a year receivables had declined by 7 days." Prior to the conversion Ken had three full-time equivalent employees (FTEs) keying claims. After conversion to a PC-based process, automated downloading of claims required the attention of one part-time employee.

Teresa Krausse, business office director at Providence Medical Center in Portland, Oregon, relates a similar experience. "We used to submit Medicaid/Welfare claims via DDE but converted to a process of downloading to a PC claims submission product in December 1991. We have lowered the time it takes to collect payment from 30 or 35 days to 10 days." Teresa noted that using DDE could result in backlogs because of fluctuations in patient volume, employee turnover, and other variations in staffing levels caused by vacations, holidays, and sick leave. The use of automated downloading eliminated those backlogs.

Additional improvements in collection experience occur when the quality of the information on the outgoing claim is improved. As mentioned earlier, after claims are downloaded from the patient accounting system into the PC, the information is "edited." Editing is a review function that performs quality control checks on the claim. At the simplest level, editing ensures that vital information such as the patient name, group number, submitted charges, or date of service is included on the claim. Logical edits act as screens for incorrectly entered claims. For example, diagnosis and procedure codes must be consistent with the patient's sex or age. Payer-specific edits may also be part of the process. Claim edit routines, by allowing on-screen revisions, eliminate clerical procedures such as retyping the claim form.

Teresa Krausse verified the improvement. "The downloading process has helped us to generate more 'clean' claims. With direct data entry, operators sporadically corrected deficiencies in claims generated by the mainframe patient accounting program. Managers had no clear record of what those deficiencies were. Error reports generated by the claims submission software quickly identify repeated problems and prompt corrections to the mainframe program."

Editing is so crucial a function that unedited claims have a much lower chance of getting paid at the time of submission. Thomas Sheibler, director of the Healthcare Transaction Network of Blue Cross of California indicated that "60 percent of unedited claims are typically returned to hospitals because of errors. Even when electronically edited and transmitted claims are rejected, hospitals are usually notified immediately, instead of days or weeks later."[3] Many vendors of patient accounting systems provide electronic claims submission. The spread of electronic claim processing is due in part to PC claims submission products and the services of electronic claim clearinghouses, discussed next.

---

[3] Elizabeth Gardner and Judith Nemes, "Hospitals Cashing In on Cleaned-Up Claims," *Modern Healthcare* (March 26, 1990), pp. 23-36.

Electronic Claim Clearinghouses

Many electronic claim submission services offer "all-payer" solutions. Their services may include printing claims. A high premium is placed on the ability to get claims to large numbers of payers electronically. This is frequently done through the services of a claim clearinghouse. Claim clearinghouses currently perform three functions:

- *They act as a post office that redistributes claims to various electronic mailboxes (they send claims to claim payers).* To perform this data transport function clearinghouses must maintain and operate a telecommunications network and support a variety of telecommunication links using different communication protocols.[4]
- *They handle translator duties, taking claims transmitted in one format and reformatting them to different payer specifications.* This reformatting function is needed when trading partners do not support EDI standards.
- *They provide edit services to providers.* Many payers have imposed rules that must be applied to electronic claims before they will accept them and these many rules complicate the exchange between payer and provider. Although some make sense, such as requiring valid data in certain fields, others are specific to certain employers or certain managed care arrangements. Clearinghouses make an effort to keep track of these payer rules to help providers ensure that claims submitted will be paid rather than rejected.

Perhaps the best known claim clearinghouse is National Electronic Information Corporation (NEIC), a company founded by major commercial insurance companies including Aetna, Travelers, John Hancock, Cigna, and Metropolitan Life. Claims are also exchanged electronically among different Blue Cross Blue Shield plans to accommodate situations in which traveling plan members

---

[4] The need for an electronic equivalent for the postal service is found throughout industries that use EDI. Although some large companies build massive telecommunications departments to provide this service, most use value added networks (VANs) to communicate with their trading partners. Claim clearinghouses can be viewed as special-purpose VANs.

receive care in the territory of another plan. There are a large number of other clearinghouse/claim submission vendors in the market.

Some providers object to having "middlemen" in the claim clearinghouses, but they perform a valuable function in making EDI work, particularly in an environment without standards. The cost of using clearinghouses has declined sharply in recent years and will decline further as standards become accepted, computer and telecommunication costs shrink, volume grows, and competition intensifies.

Despite the differing paths that electronic claims take to their final destinations, it is easier to follow a claim transmitted electronically than to track a claim sent in the mail. Unless a claim is sent via registered mail, there is no confirmation that it has been received at its intended destination. By the time a provider determines that a mailed claim has not been received by the payer, days or even weeks have been lost, and the process must start all over again. Electronically confirmed claims eliminate the disappointment felt by every collection department at the words, "We never received the claim."

The X12 standard for claims submission is called the Health Care Claim (837) and it is used by major clearinghouses such as NEIC and Medicare fiscal intermediaries. Although the process of conversion takes time, there are many payers moving to support this standard. The 837 provides one format for the transmission of many different types of claims, including among others:

- HCFA 1500 outpatient medical claims
- UB 92 inpatient hospital claims
- Dental claims
- Vision claims
- Pharmacy claims
- Home medical equipment claims
- Chiropractic claims

The advent of the 837 will provide an additional impetus to the growth of electronic claims processing because it will lower the cost of doing EDI for many participants. For providers who are already submitting claims electronically the near-term benefit will be the ability to direct claims to far more payers and reviewers such as preferred provider organizations and utilization review firms. For payers the cost of acquiring electronic claims will decrease and trading partners such as PPOs and UR firms can also transmit claims for pricing or review that are now handled via the mail.

Claim Status Inquiry

In the majority of cases claims are adjudicated within a short time and payment is made. When a claim is not paid promptly, there is usually a reason. The challenge for the patient accounting department is one of speedy problem resolution. Problem resolution may entail rounds of phone tag and the exchange of form letters in the mail. To manage the pipeline of claims in process, some providers take advantage of electronic claim status inquiry and on-line claim corrections. Teresa Krausse explains that Provident Medical Center uses an electronic claim inquiry for claims submitted to Blue Cross Blue Shield of Oregon:

> Daily lists are obtained of submitted but unpaid claims and appropriate action taken. For example, a claim may have been pending for additional information from a physician, or additional information about an accident may be needed from the patient. The staff can immediately turn to the task of acquiring that information. Claims that have been approved but not yet paid require no active follow-up, and steps can be taken to prepare for secondary billing. Follow-up procedures used to involve calling about many claims, but now calls are made on an exception basis. More timely and accurate information allows us to focus resources on problems that require resolution.[5]

In Virginia, UVAMC can obtain claim status reports about claims submitted to Medicare, Blue Cross Blue Shield, and some of the major commercial carriers. Unfortunately, many payers do not support inquiries other than by phone and mail. This will change, thanks to the recent availability of X12 EDI standards for this information exchange. Providers and payers both realize that it is expensive for both to support numerous phone calls about claims

---

[5] James J. Moynihan and Kathryn Norman, "Claims Submission Leads Electronic Advances."

in the process of adjudication. For many payers, the development of an automated inquiry and response capability was out of the question because there were no national standards and providers would only support the electronic formats used by dominant payers in each local market. ANSI X12 standards for a Health Care Claim Status Inquiry (276) and a Health Care Claim Status Response (277) will extend the benefits of electronic status inquiry across all payers.

Claim Payments

Most claim payments today are made with checks attached to paper remittance advices or explanation of benefits statements. Information available to the provider about how a payment was calculated varies in clarity and thoroughness. Not all payers have well-designed remittance forms and clear explanations of benefits statements. Unlike standardized claims forms such as the UB 92 and the HCFA 1500, no standardized forms exist for presenting remittance information to providers. Not even the terminology is standardized, because health care may be paid for by myriad insurance programs (such as group health plans, worker's compensation, auto liability, and indigent care).

For example, a patient who has insurance may be referred to as the *claimant*, the *insured*, the *member*, the *subscriber*, or the *dependent*. The lack of a standard paper format for remittance information has spawned a multitude of form designs. Information is conveyed in different terminology, found in various locations, and in differing amounts of detail on each different form. In addition, there may not be enough information anywhere to reconcile submitted charges to the paid amount.

No wonder, then, that an electronic remittance receipt has been slower to develop than the electronic claim submission. Nevertheless, the remittance receipt is attractive to providers because remittance processing and related data logging is a labor-intensive clerical task. Historically, electronic remittance information has been provided by a small percentage of payers, and it has been as unstandardized as its paper equivalent. Not many providers receive remittance information electronically for several reasons:

- It has not been widely available from payers.
- Providers prefer receiving the data accompanied by a check, because the check amount can be easily reconciled with the total remittance amount.
- Vendor support of electronic remittance transactions has been spotty.
- The electronic formats for the remittance data differ from payer to payer.
- Providers have limited data-processing staff to handle the necessary systems work.

Approval of a national standard for claims payment in the ANSI X12 format eliminates many of the barriers to widespread use of electronic remittance processing. The Health Care Claims Payment/Advice (835) can also be used in conjunction with the interbank payment system known as the Automated Clearing House (ACH) network. For providers who want funds to accompany remittance data, the ACH network can send electronic remittance data with funds. These capabilities make it possible for all providers to automate remittance processing.

Most providers wish to receive an EDI remittance file and use it to identify, post, and close the related accounts receivable with as little human intervention as possible. The cost and difficulty of doing so are systems integration issues, and the provider's vendor may not make available the necessary tools for easy, inexpensive automation.[6] Providers will also have to work with their banks if electronic funds transfers are used to replace checks. Recipients of EFT/EDI payments must be sure that their banks are EDI-capable. Banks that are not will "miss" the data sent using EFT.

No matter what degree of automation a provider chooses to process electronic remittance data, the issue of reconciling banking and accounting data sent separately must be addressed. Financial managers must bear in mind their need to reconcile the remittance data with related funds received. In a paper-based accounting environment, checks and remittance data travel together, so the recipient can visually confirm that the remittance total and the

---

[6] David F. Schinderle and James J. Moynihan, "Taming the Remittance Beast Electronically," *Healthcare Financial Management* (March 1992).

monetary total match. When electronic claims are used, the opportunity exists to have dollars and data travel separately. Providers must work with their banks to develop a collection reporting process to reassociate data and dollars that travel separately.[7]

Payers have not yet come to accept an electronic remittance advice in a secondary claim as proof of payment by the primary carrier. However, National Medical Enterprises (NME) and some other providers have effectively used the electronic remittance advice to speed up secondary billing. In some of its facilities, NME receives an electronic remittance advice from Aetna, its fiscal intermediary, and goes through the expected posting and closing routines. Information from the electronic remittance is then used to create a paper remittance advice for claims that will be sent to a secondary payer. The original invoice is retrieved from an electronic archive, printed, and attached to the remittance advice; then a new invoice is sent to the secondary carrier. This process has replaced procedures that required several days of clerical work to pull and photocopy original paper bills, photocopy the paper remittance advice, and attach both copies to a bill for the secondary payer. Today, thousands of secondary bills are ready just hours after the receipt of electronic remittance information, thus speeding cash flow and reducing labor costs.

As Medicare and additional commercial payers convert to an electronic remittance standard, electronic secondary billing should eliminate the former paper-intensive process. The timing will in part depend on how quickly providers and their vendors establish the capability to receive the electronic remittance and commit to doing business electronically. The X12 standards development process has included an effort to automate secondary billing. The Health Care Claim (837) standard can also include remittance information generated by the primary payer. Medicare fiscal intermediaries expect to use the 837 to send claim and remittance data directly to the secondary payer of record in their files. This will eliminate the provider from the work flow, lower administrative costs, and deliver payment to the provider more quickly.

---

[7] Providers should insist on using either the Corporate Trade Exchange (CTX) payment format or the CCD+ format, both of which can contain machine-readable X12 information to automate reconciliation. Additional background and detail on electronic payments can be found in Chapter 10.

Chapter Five

EDI for Managed Care

There was a time when all the transactions between payers and providers could be accommodated by standards for eligibility inquiries and responses, claim submission, claim status, and claim payments. The development of managed care has added additional transactions to the claims process, hence the need for a separate discussion of EDI for managed care.

WHAT IS MANAGED CARE?

Managed care is a term applied to many ways of administering the provision of health care. Such healthcare administration is usually explained by contrast with indemnity insurance, which has different mechanisms for controlling medical costs.

In the traditional employer-sponsored healthcare insurance arrangement, benefits were made available under an indemnity plan. Employees and their dependents selected their own healthcare providers and made their own decisions about the purchase of medical services. Employers paid insurance premiums to insurance companies that subsequently processed claims for reimbursement. Claims were submitted either by the employee or by the provider, but there was no direct contractual relationship between provider and payer. Providers were "third parties" to the payer, whose contractual relationship was with the employer and the insured. Under traditional indemnity insurance plans, payers learn about large claims after medical services are rendered. They have only a limited ability to affect costs after resources have already been expended. Some charges can be reduced if they are found to be unreasonable or not medically relevant, but such changes have little effect on the total cost of health care. The roles of the insurance company are to spread risk, prevent fraud, and administer the benefit plan.

The concept of managed care encompasses many ways of organizing and administering health care. Managed care differs from the traditional indemnity insurance by controlling the patient's access to medical services. In certain types of health maintenance organizations (HMOs), members must receive all of their care from physicians and allied health personnel employed by the HMO and in facilities owned by the HMO, with few exceptions. Managed care plans often do more than restrict access to unauthorized providers; these plans often seek to "manage the process." One example is the use of *case management*. Large cost savings can be achieved when a medical condition is managed to minimize the time the patient spends in an acute care facility. This can be done by discharging patients to skilled nursing facilities or home care as soon as the underlying medical condition allows for care in those less expensive settings. Under an indemnity plan a patient may have stayed in hospital for a longer period of time than necessary because there were limited financial incentives for the providers to reduce the length of an inpatient stay.

Utilization review (UR) is another aspect of managed care. Some medical procedures must be authorized or certified before treatment is rendered. This can be done by a UR department within a payer organization or by an independent utilization review firm. Both case management and treatment certification/authorization may reduce medical costs, but they create the need for far more transactions and information exchanges between payer and provider.

The contrast between indemnity insurance plans and managed care is no longer as great as it once was. Over time indemnity insurance plans have added additional controls. In some parts of the country such as Southern California, all private healthcare insurance incorporates some form of "managed care," and the classical indemnity insurance plan with virtually unlimited access to providers is no longer available. The hallmark of markets such as

Southern California where all care is "managed" is the extensive use of UR and treatment authorization and direct contractual relationships between payers and providers. A portion of the managed care industry also uses capitation payments to shift risk and related responsibility from the managed care company to the provider. Capitation payments are essentially premium payments made to providers that undertake the risk of providing the medical care required by members. Authorization and capitation practices in managed care have created the need for new information exchanges outside the scope of the traditional claims process. The need for these exchanges varies depending on the organizational structure of the managed care company.

ORGANIZATION OF MANAGED CARE COMPANIES

The organizational structure of firms in the managed care business varies greatly. Managed care companies may be staff-model HMOs that own hospitals, employ physicians, and also provide insurance. The staff model takes its name from the fact that physicians are "on staff" as employees. In contrast, network-model HMOs contract with dozens of hospitals and hundreds of physicians to provide the same services as the large staff-model HMOs. Healthcare providers that care for members are not employees but contractors with the HMO.

Some network-model HMOs contract with large medical groups; others contract with independent practitioner associations (IPAs) that represent physicians who are not part of a medical group. Network-model HMOs may contract with both medical groups and IPAs because the way in which medicine is organized changes a great deal from region to region. Finally, managed care services may also be provided through a variety of independent employee benefit firms working for self-insured employers. Self-insured companies want to avail themselves of the benefits of competent utilization management and retain other financial benefits from self-insurance.

Providers in these arrangements may be paid a salary, receive a prepaid fee per member per month (a *capitation payment*), or be

FIGURE 5–1
Network-model HMO data flows.

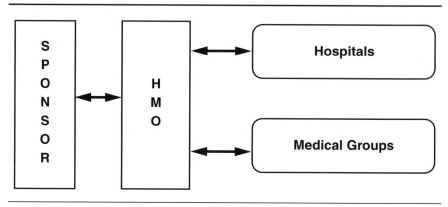

reimbursed on a fee-for-service basis with extensive utilization management. Each of these forms of managed care creates different challenges for doing business.

The information systems manager for a managed care plan that contracts with medical groups and hospitals for healthcare services has a significant challenge. That manager must deal with providers in multiple organizations, each with different computer hardware and software. All of the information about services provided to patients is collected by staff outside the plan and beyond the plan's direct control. Providers submit claims or encounter information on a variety of paper forms and, until recently, in a variety of electronic formats. The quality of coding on bills or claims varies widely and the timeliness with which information is received can be quite erratic. As a result, financial reporting is difficult. "Incurred but not reported" expenses are created when services are provided but there is a time lag before those expenditures are reported.

The Network Model

Billing and payment arrangements in managed care can be far more complex than in the indemnity world. They may include capitation payments, fee-for-service claims, and a host of contractual

FIGURE 5–2
TPA and the self-insured managed care data flows.

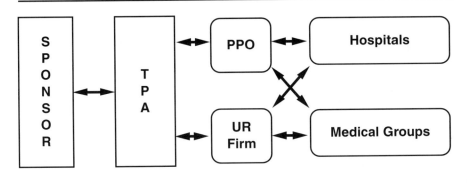

agreements. This combination of billing and payment methods is costly to administer. (Figures 5–1 shows a schematic of information gathered in this fashion.) Clearly, the informationmanager of a net-work-model HMO could benefit enormously from the use of stan-dards-based EDI to gather and transmit required information.

The Self-Insured Model

A comparable problem exists for the third-party administrator (TPA) offering case management and UR services to a self-insured employer. Some TPAs may contract for such services from a Pre-ferred Provider Organization (PPO) or a stand-alone managed care service company (see Figure 5–2) to present a complete solu-tion to an employer. These vendors compete with insurance com-panies that may have comparable departments within their orga-nizations to provide the same set of services. Those departments may be able to communicate via internal systems, but many are faced with the same communications challenges as are groups of independent vendors assembled by the self-insured employer.

The Staff Model

The comparable task of information gathering in a staff-model managed care organization (see Figure 5–3) appears easier. For an

FIGURE 5–3
Staff-model HMO data flows.

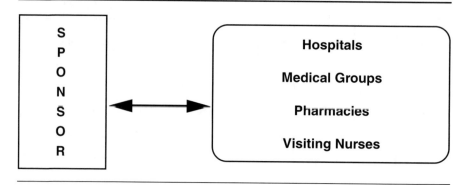

HMO that owns and operates its own hospitals and office or clinic facilities for physicians, gathering information should be easier. A centralized information systems department may collect administrative information on services provided because providers and administrators are part of a common organization and a shared information systems department. (The word *may* is used because not all staff-model organizations are automated.)

Does this mean that the staff-model HMO is inherently more efficient administratively than other managed care organizations? Perhaps, but not necessarily. If hospitals and physicians could complement their contractual linkages to payers with electronic network linkages, they could exchange information easily and slash the cost of administration. In fact, even the largest staff-model organizations have a significant need to manage the care provided by other providers. Kaiser Permanente has a sizable staff who process claims from other providers that have rendered care for Kaiser members. Network-model HMOs also reimburse "out-of-network" providers.

Collecting Encounter Data

No matter what the form of organization, managed care companies need to collect information about the services rendered to members. If they are staff-model HMOs or network-model HMOs with capitated medical groups, such information is referred to as *encounter data.* Encounter data is similar to claim data except for the absence of monetary charges. The Health Care Claim (837) was designed for use in transmitting encounter data as well as claims. Claim data from noncapitated providers or out-of-network providers will also be collected by managed care companies to track services rendered to members. Systems designed to generate invoices are found in most U.S. provider facilities, and managed care companies should be able to receive electronic encounter/claim data from providers.

The roadblock facing managed care payers seeking to use electronic claims is that many have negotiated contractual payment agreements with providers that cannot be transmitted on a standard paper form or standard EDI format. The managed care industry also has not standardized its data requirements for a standard encounter, which complicates implementation for the provider who faces varied data requirements from different payers. Within ASC X12N, representatives of managed care companies are working on a standard data set for the managed care encounter, which should facilitate EDI for encounters in the future.

Managed care companies seeking electronic claims and encounters can benefit from the significant momentum behind the market shift to electronic claims initiated by Medicare and other payers. Claims, however, are not the most important transactions to be automated in managed care. The prime candidates for automation in the managed care process are UR and referral management.

UTILIZATION REVIEW AND REFERRAL MANAGEMENT

The primary care physician is often the quarterback of the managed care referral process. Managed care plans traditionally assign a primary care physician to each patient. The primary care physician is in some ways the traditional "family doctor." In a managed care environment that physician may also be a services "gatekeeper," and one of the goals of managed care is to ensure that expensive medical specialists are used only when necessary. The process of controlling specialist utilization is called *referral management.* Administrative rules for managed care are developed for the primary care physicians, referral physicians to whom the primary care physician may send the patient for additional care, and rendering physicians who perform specialized services. These rules vary according to medical treatments and tests, and the rules change from payer to payer. In some circumstances, physicians may authorize a specialist referral within a framework laid down by the managed care company. In others, the medical group may be accepting capitation payments and develop its own internal guidelines for authorization. Authorization numbers that will be needed by the referral physician may be generated by the primary care physician, a UR firm or by the UR department of a payer. The authorization numbers granted to different providers must be tracked and checked to ensure that all necessary administrative procedures have been followed. There has been no standardization of the rules and procedures of managed care, and that has created a large administrative burden for providers who must fulfill different reporting requirements for different payers.

Failure to fulfill these requirements may mean limited or no payment to the provider by the payer and the assumption of the cost by the patient. For example, if there are a multitude of managed care organizations, hospitals can admit patients with an approval from a primary care physician and despite collecting the required authorization number, there can still be uncertainty about final payment. One physician may have contracts with several managed care plans, each of which has separate rules for when the physician can authorize additional care. In certain cases the physician may have to direct the patient to arrange some additional review process before admission. Providers report that some contracts among plans and primary care physicians are ambiguous and that interpretation by a claims examiner after the fact will determine payment.

The EDI standard designed by managed care industry representatives is the Health Services Review Report (278). According to its developers, the 278 has the potential to automate 80 percent of the authorization transactions that are handled by phone today. The authorization process currently occupies the time of thousands of nurses in both payer and provider organizations. They exchange information verbally and play phone tag. Use of the 278 transaction

FIGURE 5–4
An authorization process example among an HMO, an IPA, and a hospital not using EDI.

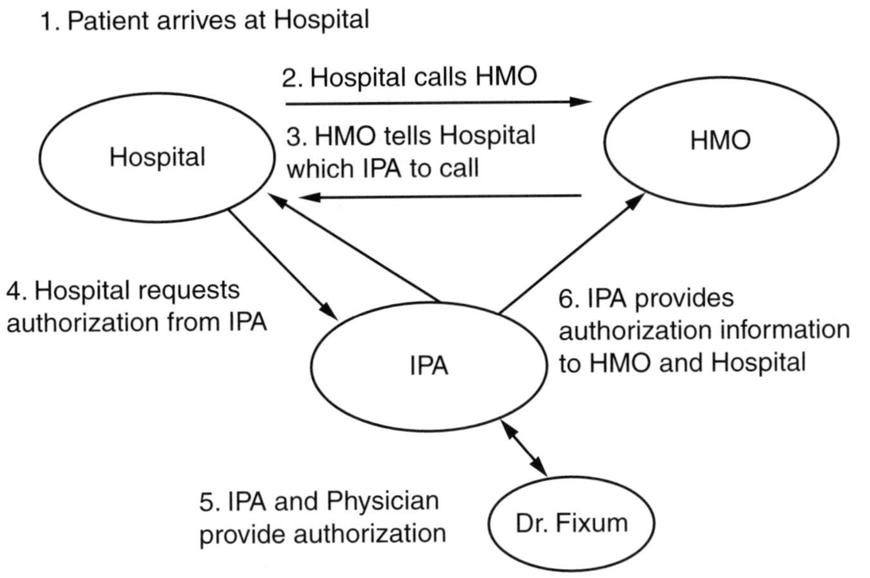

1. Patient arrives at Hospital

2. Hospital calls HMO

Hospital

3. HMO tells Hospital
which IPA to call

HMO

4. Hospital requests
authorization from IPA

IPA

6. IPA provides
authorization information
to HMO and Hospital

5. IPA and Physician
provide authorization

Dr. Fixum

will streamline the process. Two schematics in Figure 5–4 and Figure 5–5 illustrate the tremendous benefit that could accrue to payers and providers alike from use of the 278.

In Figure 5–4, the hospital learns about the patient's needs when the patient shows up at the admissions department. The patient may know the name of the referring doctor and the insurance company, but the hospital has a significant amount of investigation to perform. The HMO is usually contacted to determine whether the patient is eligible and whether the HMO or a medical group has the authority to grant an admission. The HMO can direct the hospital to the right Independent Practitioner Association (IPA), which is important because a physician may be in several IPAs with different contractual terms and authorization rules from various HMOs. The hospital must then obtain an authorization number from the IPA and be ready to submit an invoice to the

FIGURE 5–5
The authorization process example using EDI.

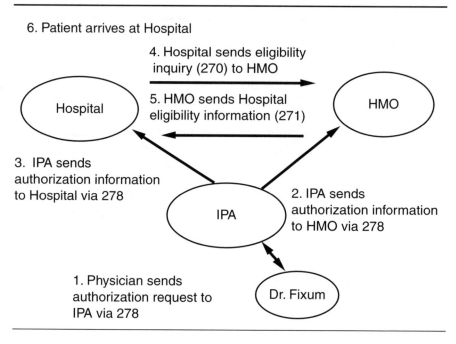

6. Patient arrives at Hospital

4. Hospital sends eligibility inquiry (270) to HMO

Hospital

5. HMO sends Hospital eligibility information (271)

HMO

3. IPA sends authorization information to Hospital via 278

IPA

2. IPA sends authorization information to HMO via 278

1. Physician sends authorization request to IPA via 278

Dr. Fixum

HMO. In a paper environment some physicians might provide a form with an authorization number that would be handed to the hospital admissions staff by the patient. Several weeks later the hospital is expected to attach that piece of paper to a claim form and send it to the HMO. Clearly this is a labor- and paper-intensive way to do business.

Figure 5–5 illustrates how EDI might be used to automate the process. Using a 278, the referring physician would initiate a request for admission authorization to the IPA staff. The IPA would authorize the admission and notify both the physician and the hospital with the 278. On receiving the 278 the hospital might still check with the HMO to determine whether the patient were currently enrolled via the 270 eligibility inquiry transaction. The HMO would transmit an eligibility response via the 271 transaction. This use of EDI would have a large impact on the admission process. The hospital would see the patient after the information had been received, resulting in these benefits:

- The patient would not have to be subjected to extensive questioning by the admission staff about sources of payment and basic demographic information, all of which would be in the 278.
- Customer service would improve because the patient could be shown to a room without the hassles of admission.
- The data the hospital obtained would also be more accurate than that obtained from the patient.
- The staff in the admitting department could be redirected to other tasks because their role of interrogating patients would be sharply reduced.

The 278 transaction is a relatively new EDI standard but its use will have a significant impact in the managed care community.

CAPITATION

Capitation has an immense impact on the use of EDI by providers and payers. Under capitated contract arrangements providers will not just submit claims, they will pay claims. Providers will become payers.

In parts of the country where managed care has a larger share of the market, major hospitals and medical groups now receive capitation payments from local HMOs. Some hospital systems and medical groups are receiving capitation payments each month for over 100,000 covered lives. This requires an entirely new administrative process for the provider's business office. The staff who undertakes responsibility for capitation contracts may not realize the administrative impact of paying for "out-of-network" care.

Here is an example: The St. Joseph Health System is an eight-hospital system based in California. Two of its hospitals are in Orange County, California, a market with a large managed care presence. SJHS has signed capitation contracts with several payers and has assumed responsibility for providing acute care services for covered members of several HMOs. Although the two hospitals are able to provide many services in-house there are services

FIGURE 5–6

The claims process with a PHO requires maintenance of two reimbursement systems based on fee-for-service claims and capitated encounters.

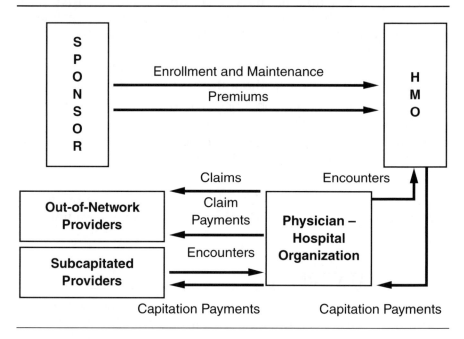

they do not offer. For example, they do not have pediatric wards, so care for children is usually provided by Orange County Children's Hospital (OCCH). Under the terms of the capitation contracts, SJHS bears financial responsibility for care rendered at the Children's Hospital. About 1,000 UB 92 bills are generated per month by OCCH and sent to the SJHS business office for payment. The business office staff has to perform functions usually fulfilled by insurance companies. They check whether the patient is covered and if the care was authorized. They review charges to see if they are in line with contracted terms. Claims are adjudicated and paid. The provider's business office has reversed its traditional role. It not only submits claims, it receives them; it not only receives payments, it makes them.

Many providers are forming physician hospital organizations (PHOs) in order to bid for capitated contracts from HMOs. This creates an administrative challenge, as illustrated in Figure 5–6. The figure illustrates how a PHO must maintain dual administrative systems and procedures. It has to track encounters or services rendered by providers at risk under the contract, as well as pay claims submitted by out-of-network providers. EDI can play an important role in the administration of managed care contracts.

MANAGED CARE ENROLLMENT

Providers in a capitated environment compete in part based on their ability to provide lower cost medical care. Cutting costs requires some changes to clinical procedures. It will also require that providers avoid providing uncompensated care for patients who are mistakenly thought to be eligible. Cutting the cost of treating patients is laudable, but capitated providers must ensure that the patient is their responsibility and not insured by some other insurance carrier. To guard against this eventuality, HMOs and capitated providers must maintain an up-to-date eligibility list. At the start of the process, the HMO should be linked electronically with the plan sponsor to manage adds, changes, and deletions. Chapter 7 describes how the Benefit Enrollment and Maintenance (834) standard can be used to establish this linkage.

The second step in the enrollment process is the transfer of an eligibility roster from the HMO to the capitated provider. Figure 5–7 illustrates this exchange, which uses the 271 Health Care Eligibility/Benefit Information standard. The crucial importance of an electronic roster is that it enables the provider to ensure that care is provided without charge only for patients who are truly eligible. Many Americans have coverage from more than one insurer, and the coordination of benefits process is vital for the provider to ensure profitability. As people change jobs, elect to accept or reject COBRA coverage, and assume responsibility for minors through divorce decrees, the determination of who is covered for health care becomes more complex. Providers that rely on piles of printed eligibility rosters that are only occasionally examined will be hard pressed to earn a profit on competitive capitation premiums.

FIGURE 5–7

Eligibility information obtained by HMOs in the 834 from sponsors is transmitted to the PHO via the eligibility information standard, the 271.

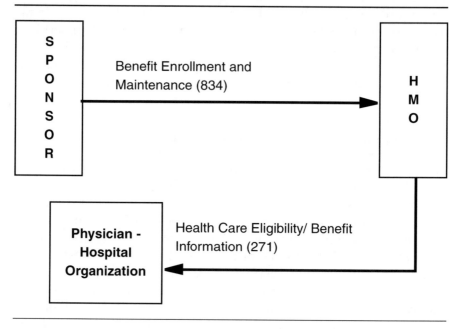

Providers need to track eligibility through two related transactions: the transmission of the eligibility roster and the capitation payment. As of mid-1995, no standard for capitation payments had emerged from the ASC X12N subcommittee, but a workgroup has made progress on such a standard. Capitation payments will likely be made electronically through the use of the 835 Health Care Claim Payment/Remittance Advice standard first approved in 1991 that is widely used for the payment of Medicare claims.

PROVIDERS AS PAYERS

In addition to the use of managed care transactions such as those for authorization (278) and eligibility roster transmission (271), providers in a capitated contract can use the EDI standards for claims (837) and claims payments (835). The St. Joseph Health System (SJHS) described earlier traditionally transmitted electronic claims and received claim payments. In its new role as a claim payer, it realized it could slash processing costs by receiving electronic claims from out-of-network providers and by paying those providers electronically. In order to obtain electronic claims, SJHS became the first provider in the country to be issued an NEIC payer ID number. Other providers will follow suit and turn to their claim submission vendors for claims receipt services as well as claim transmission services.

As is true for insurance companies, providers can realize significant benefits from receiving electronic claims. The largest cost of administering claim processing is labor, and the largest single component of labor is the claims data entry and examination function. The productivity available from electronic claims receipt and autoadjudication is dramatic. Claim examiners who once processed 60 claims an hour can approve 160 claims an hour after implementation of electronic claims receipt. That translates into lower staffing requirements. Providers are in a good position to work with clearinghouses and other providers to do business electronically. The longer-term goals should be to implement EDI throughout the claims process. The claims adjudication systems acquired should support EDI eligibility inquiries and responses as well as electronic claims payments. In some states, such as Arizona, providers acting as payers may be subject to legislation that requires electronic capabilities for claims processing.

Finally, providers that become payers under capitated contracts must be prepared to pay healthcare claims electronically. The solution chosen by the SJHS mentioned in this chapter is worth retelling. The health system chose to outsource its claims payments to its bank. A file is transmitted in the 835 format to the bank which pays EDI-capable providers electronically. Non-EDI-capable providers receive a check and an explanation of benefit statement printed and mailed by the bank. This solution allowed the health system to avoid investment in printing capabilities for EOBs in a limited production environment. It also automated exchanges with EDI-capable providers to lower overall operating expenses.

Chapter Six

EDI for Procurement

America's healthcare providers are reengineering the procurement process, and EDI is playing a vital role. Previously, reimbursement methods were "charge-based" and materials managers paid a great deal of attention to accurate "charge capture" systems. If an item was used but not charged to the patient's account, the provider could not be reimbursed. Inventory management during this period was not focused on inventory reduction; rather, the concern was the consequence of running out of a product or supply, which in health care could be life-threatening. In this era, physicians were free to use the products or supplies they chose, without consultation with their colleagues. This could result in the use, and maintenance in inventory, of six almost identical suture materials from six different manufacturers being used by six surgeons. For these reasons, the inventory levels at many hospitals were often excessive. The transition to a more competitive environment, including fixed price payments and lower profit margins, has resulted in major changes. "Just-in-time" concepts are replacing "just-in-case" practices.

The hospital materials management professional has far more in common with a material management specialist in other industries than is generally the case for other healthcare professions. The process diagrammed in Figure 6–1 can be applied equally to a hospital or a manufacturing firm. Many of the best ideas in purchasing and distribution management in industry can generally be found in the professional literature of hospital material managers.

FIGURE 6–1
EDI standards for the procurement process can be readily adopted in the healthcare industry.

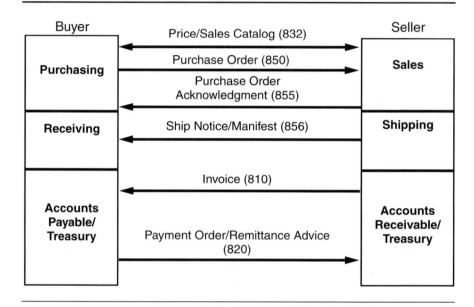

Although every hospital has unique priorities, broad generalizations about the steps taken to cut costs can be listed:

- *Group Purchasing:* If a hospital was not already part of a group purchasing organization, it joined one to get better contract prices from the major suppliers.
- *Vendor Consolidation:* Many hospitals directed their purchasing dollars to distributors rather than buying direct from manufacturers. In addition, the number of distributors used was reduced as providers developed either "prime vendor" or "sole distributor" relationships.
- *Inventory Item Reduction:* Although it is often difficult to change physician preferences, efforts have been made to standardize inventory items.
- *Reduced Inventory Levels:* The gospel of "just-in-time" inventory management has spread through the ranks of hospital material managers. When possible, providers have turned to

their distributors to assume the warehousing function formerly filled by a storage facility on or near the provider site. The trade-off has been more frequent deliveries from the distributor. The ability to eliminate on-site inventory varies greatly from hospital to hospital, depending on location, weather and physical plant. Remote snowbound hospitals or city hospitals with small delivery docks obviously cannot achieve the same success with this kind of program as hospitals situated close to their distributor or hospitals with more spacious receiving docks in better locations. Well-situated hospitals have developed "stockless purchasing" programs with their distributor making deliveries to individual departments within the hospital.

THE IMPACT ON FINANCE

Healthcare financial managers are usually responsible for the final steps in the purchase process. The finance organization customarily handles the receipt of invoices and then generates related vendor payments. The accounts payable department that handles these tasks is obviously part of the total procurement process. Purchasing and accounts payable are two departments that frequently report to different managers and sometimes seem to operate with different agendas. Communication is sometimes lacking between the two, but neither department can operate in isolation.

When material managers opt for a restocking program with their prime vendor, the number of invoices may increase six-fold. Planning must be coordinated between the two departments and the historical separation of the accounts payable and materials management departments must be reexamined.

THE TRADITIONAL PURCHASING OPERATION

The separation of the accounts payable and the purchasing functions is traditional, because of audit and control issues. The rationale has been that those who are given the authority to purchase goods should be separated from those who pay for those purchases to prevent collusion. The logic of departmental separation was reinforced in the days before computers. The purchasing department managed the ledger cards that kept track of the warehouse. The accounts payable department managed the "tickets" that fed the general ledger system. The purchasing department replenished the warehouse at intervals that would not overwhelm the payables department with transactions. The *economic order quantity (EOQ)* algorithm was developed to balance the transaction costs of acquisition with the capital costs of holding inventory and the discounts available for bulk purchases. Healthcare financial managers are still taught the EOQ model today as it was taught when introduced before World War I. In the interim, revolutionary changes occurred in the communication and transportation industries.

New managerial approaches, usually referred to as just-in-time inventory management, have proven more successful than traditional models. Healthcare financial managers, like their counterparts in other industries, are learning that the supply acquisition process can be radically improved. In order to do so, procurement must be examined in a new light. The impact on the accounts payable staff may be radical. Some companies have substituted electronic invoices for paper transactions, but others have eliminated the use of invoices altogether. Similarly, some companies have substituted electronic funds transfers for checks for a major portion of their vendors. Other innovations include outsourcing the printing of checks and remittance advices as well as the use of corporate credit cards called *procurement cards*.

Although each transaction automated can be beneficial, the best strategic goal is to use EDI to improve and reengineer the procurement process. Providers can use EDI to reduce the total cost of supplies, and healthcare financial managers can guide other managers to a better understanding of the costs and benefits involved.

EVALUATING SUPPLY EXPENSES

Healthcare financial managers who have studied the potential savings from EDI applications realize that current financial reporting procedures for balance sheet and income statement presentations are misleading. Most nonprofit hospitals understate inventory values on their balance sheets. Unfortunately, that may mean that management may underestimate the large amount of capital tied up in inventory-related costs for handling and obsolescence. Does management set specific goals for inventory turnover and days of supply on hand and monitor those statistics frequently?

In contrast, financial managers in the accounts receivable department are instructed to meet target levels of "days in accounts receivable." In fact, the dollar amount of inventory shown on many provider balance sheets is misleading. Many providers differentiate between "official" and "unofficial" inventories, that is, nonstock items. This accounting practice has a major impact. Hospital providers may have unofficial inventory that is 10 times greater than official inventory. Financial analysis of a typical provider's accounts may indicate that annual inventory turnover (total supply expense/year-end inventory) appears to be 6 times a year. Thus end-of-the-year inventory on hand is equal to a 60-day supply. In fact, when unofficial inventory is estimated and included in the calculation, inventory turnover is less than once a year and ending inventory appears to be in excess of a year's supply. How much of this inventory is obsolete or overstocked?

Financial reporting procedures for the income and expense statement also understate the financial impact of supply expense. Financial managers are acutely aware that labor expense is the single largest provider expense; supply expense follows as a distant second. Supply expense is understated because it includes only the *acquisition cost* and none of those costs incurred up until the point of use. In a manufacturing enterprise, raw materials are acquired, and the labor resources expended are added to the work in progress account. Only at the time of sale is the related inventory charged as an expense. Imagine the impact on the financial statement of allocating all the labor of materials management, nurses, and physicians incurred during a hip joint replacement procedure to the value of the surgical supplies used in the procedure. Supply expense would appear to be vastly greater.

This comparison between provider and manufacturing expense calculations is not made to urge providers to adopt complicated costing procedures for inventory reporting. The point is that the magnitude of the resources dedicated to the acquisition and use of supplies is far greater than the financial statements indicate.

FIGURE 6–2
Components in a "revalued" estimate of total supply costs. **(Reprinted courtesy of Baxter Healthcare.)**

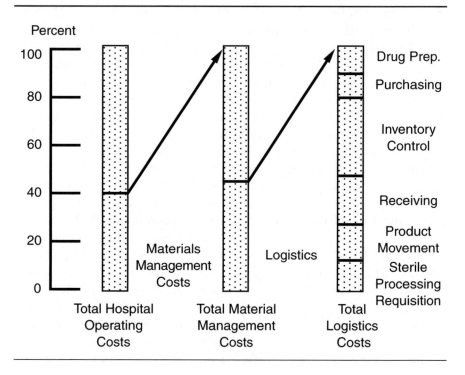

Figure 6–2 illustrates how logistics and transaction expenses combine with acquisition cost to produce a total cost of supplies that far exceeds what appears on the income statement. Logistical expenses are added to the base purchase price for a total cost of acquisition.

Healthcare financial managers may not accept these estimates for total supply expenses, but whatever the final number for any individual facility, the chief financial officer or the controller and accounting staff of a hospital bear the responsibility for the administrative costs of purchasing and accounts payable. In an unautomated environment the acquisition process generates significant costs and mountains of paper. The following discussion is taken from a presentation by Thomas Pirelli, CEO of Enterprise Systems, at an American Society of Hospital Material Managers annual meeting. It conveys the urgency of automating these transactions.

PURCHASE ORDER CONSIDERATIONS

Typically, hospital purchase orders (POs) are preprinted, four- or five-part carbon (or NCR paper) forms made to be filled out on a typewriter or computer printer. Some hospitals print as many as seven copies of each PO, each copy color-coded for a specific purpose, such as:

Copy 1: Vendor Copy

Copy 2: Purchasing Copy

Copy 3: Accounting Copy

Copy 4: Receiving Copy

Copy 5: Receiving Copy (for back-orders)

Copy 6: Department Confirmation Copy

Copy 7: Department Confirmation Copy (for second department)

This archaic process wastes trees, valuable file space, and time consumed in bursting, collating, and filing all that paper.

Why Use Paper at All?

With today's computer technology, hospital purchase orders can be created and sent to vendors, be compared with items received, initiate payment of invoices, and be permanently archived without ever using a piece of paper in the process. Eliminating paper represents major cost savings—even after deducting the cost of the laser disk storage units that replace the paper and filing cabinets. These units are called *CD-WORMS (compact disk-write once, read many storage)*. A typical hospital purchase order for 10 medical supply items contains approximately 1,000 characters of information. A CD-WORMS unit for an inexpensive personal computer can store 650 million characters of information. This means that a single removable disk the size of an audio CD can store approximately 650,000 purchase orders.

Number of Purchase Order Copies

How many purchase orders does a hospital generate per year? Even if a facility produces 60,000 POs per year, it could store 10 years' worth on a single CD. Think of all the expensive filing space consumed by the paper for 60,000 POs. In addition, most hospitals do not store just one copy of each PO. Multiple receiving copies stapled to packing slips, department copies, accounting copies, purchasing copies, and so on, are all filed away in hospital filing cabinets, taking up an enormous amount of space.

Accounting Considerations

What happens when the accounts payable department receives a copy of a purchase order? The staff waits for an invoice to come in. Do they then pay on that invoice? No, they wait to receive another copy of the PO, in the form of a receiving document that verifies that the items were received. This means that the accounts payable department has now collected four pieces of paper to process a single purchase order: the original PO, the receiving copy, the packing slip, and the vendor's invoice. When all four pieces of paper match perfectly, the clerks create another piece of paper, the payment voucher. Accounts payable file cabinets are overflowing with five times as much paper as the purchasing file cabinets. This purchase process is illustrated in Figure 6–3.

A purchase transaction may start life as a departmental requisition that becomes a purchase order to a vendor or distributor. Many hospitals use an electronic purchase order/electronic order entry product of some sort,[1] but usually the purchasing department clerk rekeys data from the requisition and prints a copy of

---

[1] Trading partners began electronic purchasing communications years ago by keying POs into Bell Teletype terminals. American Hospital Supply—now part of Baxter Healthcare—developed the ASAP program, now widely used as ASAP Express. Other similar products are Johnson and Johnson's Coact and Abbott Labs' Quicklink. Some group purchasing organizations offer EDI software; it is also available within material management systems that combine EDI with inventory management functions. The EDI adoption scenario in health care is following that in other industries: generic standards are developed, after which proprietary networks are abandoned. For healthcare material management applications, this move to open standards is under the auspices of the Health Information Business Communications Council (HIBCC).

FIGURE 6–3

In most hospitals in the mid-1990s, most transactions other than purchase orders and confirmations are processed using paper.

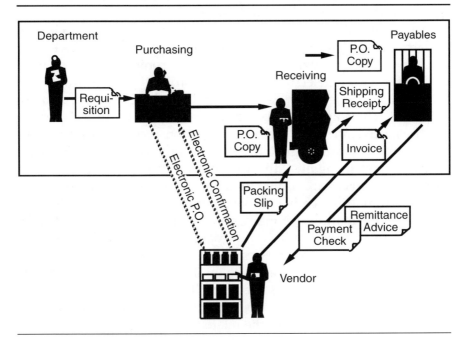

what was transmitted electronically. The transmission of electronic purchase orders in this fashion is an isolated automated act among many paper-based transactions.

The product information on the purchase order is received by the vendor into its order entry system and is used to generate a "pick ticket" to fill the order. The same information is placed on shipping documents and captured by the buyer's receiving area. The receiving area compares the information on the shipping documents with the purchase order and, if they match, both are sent on to the accounts payable department.

After making the shipment, the vendor generates an invoice reusing the same product information that appeared on all the other documents. The accounts payable department of the buyer receives the invoice and compares it with the purchase order and receiving documents. If there is a three-way match, payment is authorized.

The EDI approach to this process is to electronically exchange the required information at every point in the purchase process, from the initial departmental requisition to the final vendor payment. Figure 6–4 illustrates how this works.

Departmental requisitions are routed through the purchasing department and, when items are not filled from existing inventory stock, a purchase order is transmitted electronically to the vendor or distributor. The electronic purchase order is processed through the vendor's order entry system, and products are selected for shipment. The shipment is barcoded so that the provider's receiving area need not enter data. Information recorded through the barcode reader can be matched by the provider's material management system against the original electronic purchase order. Electronic invoices are transmitted by the vendor to the purchaser. The electronic invoice is compared with the purchase order and shipping information using a computer application; in most cases this is a feature of the accounts payable program. If there is a three-way match an accounts payable action is created.

The next step in the process is to initiate an EDI vendor payment. An EDI payment combines electronic funds transfer between the buyer's and the vendor's banks with the information necessary for the vendor to post and close the related accounts receivable.

REENGINEERING PROCUREMENT

Healthcare providers can reengineer the procurement process to help meet their expense reduction goals. EDI and a variety of other electronic commerce tools can be used to eliminate errors and transactions throughout the process. Healthcare financial managers may not have much interest in electronic purchase orders, but the accounts payable function cannot be isolated from purchasing procedures. Errors cannot be reduced without cooperation among vendors, the material management department, and the accounts payable department. In many accounts payable departments, up to one in four invoices contains a discrepancy with purchase orders that requires investigation and resolution. The elimination of errors in the invoice matching process is one of the key first steps for implementing EDI in the procurement process. Many of those discrepancies occur because the prices in the buyer's files have not

FIGURE 6–4

Hospitals that adopt EDI and electronic commerce can automate all of the major transactions as illustrated through standards-based EDI, EFT, and barcoding.

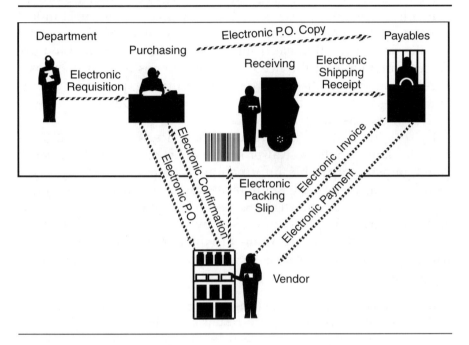

been updated. The solution is to use EDI notification of price updates. The specific EDI standard for this purpose is called the Price Sales/Catalog (832). Use of the 832 can automatically update files in a timely manner.[2]

---

[2] Most vendors have not made electronic price updates available to healthcare providers, because providers were not ready to receive them. Providers in turn did not become prepared to receive the information because vendors did not send it, creating a "chicken-and-egg" problem common in the adoption of new technologies. Today, group purchasing organizations that represent a great deal of purchasing power are demanding that vendors support electronic price update transactions, and vendors have learned that providers will be installing EDI capability for claims applications that will work for purchases as well.

Kaiser Permanente of Southern California is one healthcare provider that understands the importance of the price catalog update to improve its procurement process. They realized that it makes little sense to repeatedly transmit prices on purchase orders that differ from the prices sent back on invoices. Jerry Huntley, director of accounting, sums it up. "We want to work with our suppliers to ensure that electronic invoices can be matched to purchase orders without the need for debit memos or the other costs of resolving mismatches. Our data about pricing, product descriptions and sales tax must match that of our suppliers or we will both bear the costs of error resolution."

Kaiser's first step was to request the Price Sales/Catalog (832) from its key suppliers. Kaiser's staff then analyzed the pricing data against comparable information in their materials management purchasing system. Regular meetings were held with suppliers to review the findings. Some discrepancies resulted from data-entry errors by the suppliers or by Kaiser. Others were attributable to varying interpretations of which items were taxable and which were not. The process yielded immediate benefits. According to Huntley,

> It took some time and some changes in procedures on our part and on the part of our suppliers, but the results have been dramatic. Matching errors with one supplier declined by 90 percent. That eliminated a great deal of work and added to the success of our electronic commerce program. We have been able to reduce labor costs substantially, largely due to EDI and better relationships with our largest suppliers.

Kaiser and other progressive providers started their EDI implementation program with an emphasis on the 832 to eliminate errors. They wisely realized that receipt of electronic invoices would serve little purpose if the three-way matching process could not be automated because of mismatches between purchase orders and invoices. Once mismatches were eliminated, receipt of electronic invoices from their key vendors would eliminate the labor of keying in thousands of documents. Most providers are already sending electronic purchase orders because their material managers have implemented EDI to speed up delivery of goods. The addition of the electronic price catalog standard (832) and the electronic invoice (810) are the next steps to reducing costs through EDI.

It is likely that a provider requesting electronic invoices from a vendor will be faced with a request for a reciprocal electronic payment. Some concern about updating the payment function stems from worries about loss of float in making vendor payments. Electronic funds transfers are covered in depth in Chapter 10, but one point should be stressed here. Paying electronically is not an issue of *when* payment is made but *how* it is made. Electronic payments can be scheduled to achieve "float-neutral payment." The new opportunity is for the provider to take discounts that are currently unavailable because it takes too long to process the paperwork.

Many hospital chief financial officers (CFOs) might express little support for paying vendors electronically until they are reimbursed electronically. In most hospitals the focus in finance is on the accounts receivable function. Now that HCFA has adopted the X12 standard for electronic claims payment, the Health Care Claim Payment/Advice (835), providers can apply EDI to payment processing for both collections and disbursements. The electronic mailbox that receives electronic remittance information from a payer can also be used for receipt of electronic invoices. The EDI software that can process electronic purchase orders and invoices can be used for remittance processing as well. An EDI-capable bank can provide further economies by automating EDI vendor payments. The impetus for adopting all of these EDI exchanges lies in the ability to substantially cut costs. Providers may slash costs by eliminating 50 percent or more of the invoices and checks they process today.

EDI PLUS PROCUREMENT CARDS: THE WINNING COMBINATION

The use of EDI standards for catalog updates, purchase orders, invoices, and payments can eliminate transaction processing costs and errors. Providers can benefit from automating all of these transactions with their key EDI-capable vendors. To eliminate more paper and related costs, vendors that are not EDI-capable should be requested to supply their products through the key distributors chosen by the provider. These two steps should be accompanied by a program to shift a third class of vendors to the use of corporate procurement cards.

Although EDI is appropriate for medical and pharmaceutical suppliers, many transactions between providers and suppliers never involve a purchase order and cannot generate an electronic invoice. The challenge for financial managers is how to pay for low-cost purchases. The processing cost for these items today is quite high. An example will prove the point.

In one large multihospital system, local doughnut shops are instructed to send invoices to the centralized accounts payable operation. When the invoices are received, a voucher form is attached and sent in the interoffice mail to the requesting department. The voucher form has to be signed by the appropriate department supervisor and returned to central purchasing for further review by the accounts payable staff. (In some operations the voucher signed by the department supervisor has to include a list of all present at the event where the doughnuts were consumed.) Sometimes the name and address of the doughnut shop have to be entered as a new vendor in the accounts payable system. Even if the shop is an established vendor, several reviews by accounts payable staff occur as part of the normal accounting department checks and balances. Finally, a check and remittance advice are produced and mailed. Later, the check will be reconciled and filed away.

The obvious question is, how much did those doughnuts actually cost? With the costs associated with setting up a vendor on the system, obtaining departmental approvals, and processing accounts payable reviews, has it cost $100 to process a payment for $25 worth of doughnuts!

The problem of paying for low-cost items faces most businesses. A recent analysis by the Office of Management and Budget for the State of Ohio found that 65 percent of total approval vouchers were for under $1,000 and they accounted for only 1 percent of the dollar volume. The State of Ohio and many corporations are turning to procurement cards, a new automated solution that uses EDI but also incorporates the payment mechanisms of the credit card processing system. Procurement cards are also called *corporate puchasing cards,* and they are issued by a number of banks. Cards are given to each department within a company and an individual within each department is given the responsibility for card usage. Vendors are asked to accept credit card payment instead of traditional checks. If they are willing to do so, they receive payment immediately and do not have to submit an invoice and wait until a check is cut. The corporate buyer receives one consolidated invoice in place of hundreds—if not thousands—of individual invoices. Unlike consumer credit cards, corporate cards have additional controls:

- Dollar limits can be set by department or by individual users within a department.
- There can be restrictions on the frequency of use within a certain time period.
- Some card issuers even allow buyers to restrict use of the card to industries within certain SIC codes. For example, a card could be used by an engineering division for hardware store acquisitions but not for entertainment and travel expenses.

Companies using procurement cards can receive all the data available on purchase transactions in an electronic format. This EDI application enables the buyer to enter transaction data into internal systems for post-purchase audit and review by the appropriate approval process. Update of relevant journal and general ledger accounts can be automated. Some vendors include reporting purchases from unincorporated suppliers that can be a prelude to the generation of Form 1099 at the end of the year. As this business grows, vendors will offer more and more analytical services based on the mountains of data available from electronic processing. Information lost in a blizzard of invoices can be analyzed when captured through the electronic billing process. Electronic invoices from the card issuer can replace thousands of invoices, and hospitals can pay the card issuer by a single electronic payment that will replace thousands of checks.

IS THE ACCOUNTS PAYABLE DEPARTMENT STILL NECESSARY?

During the 1980s American automotive manufacturers used EDI to automate most of their purchase transactions. They realized that the invoice no longer served any real purpose. The logic of the automakers was simple: If the information on the invoice or receiving document about the shipment received matched the purchase order, what new information did the invoice provide? The purchase order contained the pricing and underlying contracts (such as terms of payment). As a result the auto companies now practice evaluated receipt settlement, in which payment is initiated after receipt of goods rather than after receipt of invoices. EDI audit controls are used to ensure that payments are made according to contractual terms.

In time this practice may spread to healthcare providers and their distributors. Senior financial mangers have an equal opportunity to simplify their procedures and possibly to reengineer their organizations.

Chapter Seven

EDI for the Human Resource Department

Employers and other healthcare plan sponsors, who pay the ultimate bill for healthcare costs, play a crucial role in the EDI exchanges that take place in the U.S. healthcare system. Such sponsors—be they employers, unions, or government agencies—design benefit plan contracts that are administered by insurance companies and benefit administrators. The term *plan sponsors* covers various entities that play a common role in the healthcare process. The terms of the benefit contract and the accuracy of the list of enrolled, covered individuals have a large impact on the claim process. This is true regardless of whether the plan sponsor is an employer, a government agency, or a Taft-Hartley union plan. If plan sponsors do not communicate additions or deletions to their list of covered lives in a timely manner, the benefit administrator will respond incorrectly to eligibility inquiries and adjudicate claims incorrectly. If the quality of the claim process is to be improved errors must be removed from the process at its origin where the master list of covered individuals is maintained.

This chapter describes EDI applications for the employer that can also be used by other types of plan sponsors. For larger employers that provide healthcare benefits for their employees the master list of covered individuals is maintained by the human resource department. Although applications of EDI and electronic commerce are new to the human resource department, significant opportunities have already arisen to cut costs and improve services.

Two EDI standards have been designed specifically for use by the human resource (HR) department. Their use, together with additional applications of electronic commerce, can provide significant immediate savings for employers. Some employers have used interactive voice-response software, and automated time and attendance systems to eliminate clerical tasks. An X12 EDI standard, Benefit Enrollment and Maintenance (834), can be used to electronically transmit enrollment data to benefit administrators. Another EDI standard, First Report of Injury (148) can be used to report work-related injuries to workers' compensation carriers and state agencies. These applications can reduce staff levels in the human resource department and lower the cost of employee benefits. The greatest gains will accrue to employers that work with their benefit administrators to revamp and expand the enrollment process. New procedures and the use of EDI can tighten controls on eligibility and reduce the cost of employee benefits.

EMPLOYEE COMPENSATION AND ADMINISTRATIVE EXPENSE

The cost of employee compensation is a combination of the cost of payroll and benefit programs, and the administrative expenses (both internal and external) of providing benefits. Much has been written about the cost of benefits for employees, but less has been explored about the administrative costs of providing employee benefits. The goal of efficient human resource administration is to ensure that as many dollars as possible spent on employee benefits are received by employees rather than wasted in administrative overhead. This is not a trivial issue. Healthcare costs are driving the increase in the costs of many benefit programs, and administrative overhead uses a large portion of each dollar spent for health care. Most studies do not even consider the administrative overhead incurred by the corporate employer.

Corporate employers need to be aware of their own internal administrative costs. If payroll and human resource department overhead is added to the fees charged by all the benefit administrators, the resulting figure can be used to calculate the total administrative expense per employee for the organization. That figure may vary widely from one company or industry to another, but the use of EDI can reduce those costs as illustrated by the experience of companies cited in this chapter. The human resource department should be adopting a strategy to improve the benefit administration process with a measurable goal of reducing the administrative costs of employee benefits as previously calculated. This type of process improvement is the ultimate goal of EDI.

PROCESS IMPROVEMENT

The HR department can benefit from the lessons learned by successful companies that have improved quality, increased productivity, and achieved faster turnaround times. The success stories illustrate common strategies:

- Successful companies seek to be partners, rather than adversaries, with their vendors.
- Partnership relations are cemented by electronic linkages that allow vital business information to be transmitted from computer-to-computer without mail delays and data entry errors.
- Automation of data exchange is accompanied by steps to improve the process of how trading partners do business. The business process is simplified, data exchange is automated, and related systems are integrated.

The challenge for human resource professionals is to identify their business process and then simplify, automate, and integrate the business transactions for that process.

THE INCREASING WORKLOAD FOR THE HUMAN RESOURCES DEPARTMENT

Why are the costs of administering the payroll and human resource functions increasing so significantly? Employee benefit programs are becoming more complex and expensive to administer. Employees are now faced with a large array of benefit programs for insurance and retirement needs. "Cafeteria-style" benefit plans, offered by an increasing number of employers, enable employees to customize their benefit options. The problem with tremendous variety and endless customization options is that they create additional administrative costs for the employer. The process of collecting all this information from employees and disseminating it to the appropriate benefit administrators is expensive. New developments in technology and new insights about the process can simplify benefit administration and lower benefit costs. A number of pioneers have automated the collection and dissemination of the information used for payroll and benefit administration to achieve major savings. The result has been a decrease in the staffing required for the human resource department and significant reductions in the cost of some benefit programs, particularly healthcare benefits.

WHAT IS THE PROCESS FOR THE HUMAN RESOURCE DEPARTMENT?

The two main processes that are the responsibility of the HR department are

- Benefit administration
- Payroll

Not all of the transactions related to payroll and benefit administration are handled internally. The typical human resource department relies heavily on external vendors. Healthcare claims are usually paid by third-party administrators or insurance companies; pension administration is handled by a variety of specialists; and even payroll is frequently administered by vendors. Despite outsourcing much of the processing work, the HR department is burdened with clerical tasks. These stem from the day-to-day administration of enrollment and benefit selection, as well as the collection of time and attendance data.

Benefit Administration

Information obtained when employees enroll or select benefits must be transmitted to various benefit administrators. Healthcare-related data may go to an insurance company or to a third-party administrator (TPA). Pension-related choices are sent to

FIGURE 7–1
Employers that gather benefit selection information and related periodic payroll deduction information must disseminate that data to many benefit administrators.

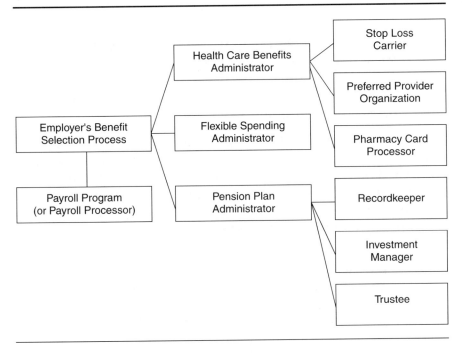

pension administrators, and information about insurance products is sent to the relevant vendor. If enrollment is inaccurate or if the information is transmitted to trading partners in an untimely fashion, all the related billing and payment transactions will be subject to error. Figure 7–1 illustrates the linkage between benefit selection and other trading partners by one employer using a variety of outside vendors for benefit processing.

Benefit selection has an important impact on the payroll process. Deductions from wages are determined by the benefit selections made by the employee. The resulting payroll deductions give rise to many other transactions. Information and funds must be transferred to insurance carriers, government agencies, and benefit administrators. The clerical work related to this process depends on the size of the work force and current procedures, but most employers would benefit from automation.

CASE STUDIES OF EDI USES IN HUMAN RESOURCE FUNCTIONS

The Bergen Brunswig Experience: Automate and Integrate Enrollment

Bergen Brunswig is a $4 billion per annum distributor of pharmaceutical products, with 4,000 employees in 40 locations throughout the United States. Larry Black is the director of compensation and benefits, and under his direction the human resource department has adopted EDI principles and practices that have been used by the company for other applications for many years.

Larry explains,

> Bergen Brunswig is a recognized industry leader in the use of EDI. We have built and expanded electronic linkages with our suppliers and our customers over the years, and have applied the basic principles to the human resource function to cut our administrative costs.

One of the first principles of process improvement is to identify the business cycle and the transactions in the cycle. Automation is best implemented at the start of the process where errors will create problems throughout. Bergen Brunswig began its application of EDI in the right place, the beginning of the process, in the HR department:

> The workload in our human resource department had increased as our benefit plan options became more complex. The enrollment of new employees took more time and benefit selection involved numerous forms. The information on the forms then had to be entered into our HR system and used to update our payroll system. It took many people a lot of time to complete these repetitive tasks. Our solution was to apply the classic EDI approach, automate data capture when possible and eliminate all redundant key entry. First, we installed a voice response system that allowed employees to enter their own benefit selections via Touch-Tone phone. Then we fed that information

into the HR system and the payroll system. New employees are first assigned a payroll number and they can then make benefit selections through the voice response product. These applications have allowed us to reduce the staffing level of our Compensation Benefits and Payroll Department from 21 to 17 in 18 months.

Automated Recording of Timekeeping and Attendance for Payroll

Another application of electronic commerce for the human resource department is automated time and attendance taking for payroll purposes. Automated data acquisition is widely used by hospitals for timekeeping and attendance systems. This situation has evolved because hospitals make extensive use of part-time employees and even the full-time employees may work different shifts.

Companies such as API and Kronos have installed their hardware and software in many hospitals, demonstrating substantial savings. The first step in automated timekeeping and attendance is the replacement of the paper timecard and/or paper timesheet. ID cards with magnetic stripes are scanned by card readers that capture the information on the card. The information gathered can be transferred to the payroll system or an external payroll processor. As is the case with so many EDI applications, the benefits extend beyond the mere elimination of data-entry tasks.

"Under the previous [paper-based] system supervisors never had the opportunity to review payroll until after it had been paid. [Now] they can review attendance in terms of tardiness and how overtime is occurring. They'd never been able to do this before," explained Brigid Hall, director of personnel at Asbury-Salina Regional Medical Center in Salina, Kansas.

Time and attendance data gathered for payroll purposes will also have an impact on the work done by benefit administrators. For example, flexible spending administrators will pay claims submitted by employees up to the amount available from related payroll deductions. Information from the payroll program (or the payroll processor) is needed to maintain the records of the flexible spending administrator or else claims will be paid in error. Employees who are paid by a worker's compensation carrier after an injury or who take a leave of absence may not make the normal

FIGURE 7–2

Flexible spending administrators require enrollment information from an employer as well as payroll information.

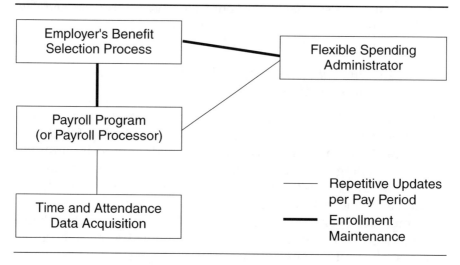

repetitive contribution to various payroll deductions. Although the process may differ for each benefit vendor that relies on payroll deductions, there is usually a ripple effect whenever there are changes in payroll deductions. Figure 7–2 illustrates the linkages between payroll and flexible spending administration.

FROM AUTOMATED DATA ACQUISITION TO EDI

Automated timekeeping and attendance data as well as electronic benefit selection offer quick short-term returns in improved efficiency. More can be done with EDI after these initial steps. Employers that acquire enrollment data electronically not only can update their own systems readily but also update those of their trading partners using EDI.

Until recently Bergen Brunswig exchanged little information with its benefit administrators electronically, in part because there were no national standards for sending that information:

In the past, we provided our health benefits administrator with a magnetic tape containing enrollment data but information exchanges with our 401K plan administrator were all done on paper. We incur substantial costs because this is not done electronically. The administrative charges for 401K administration are significant, especially because employees may change investment options, and any change will result in a cascade of paper transactions, as we notify the administrator, who notifies the investment manager, who notifies the trustee bank, and we all adjust our accounting systems. We plan to communicate these changes electronically and expect our administrators to do the same so that costs can be reduced throughout the process.

The human resources professional who uses a payroll processing firm can enjoy the same benefits. Payroll processors would vastly prefer to obtain information in an electronic format rather than process paper-based instructions. Substantial costs could be eliminated if information could be received electronically rather than by mail or fax.

HOW IMPORTANT IS EDI ENROLLMENT?

EDI transmissions usually benefit the receiver more than the sender. There are usually immediate savings available to the receiver of an electronic transmission because all the data entry work has been eliminated. Benefit administrators will certainly be able to cut costs through receipt of electronic enrollment data, and the corporate employers that send the data will pay fewer claims. The benefits of eliminating data entry costs for the benefits administrator are vastly exceeded by the savings in reduced claim expenses for the employer.

Why does EDI enrollment result in lower claim expenses? Without updated enrollment data, health benefit administrators may pay ineligible claims. One of the first American companies to use the EDI standard for electronic enrollment was AT&T. That company now transmits electronic enrollment data to its claim administrators. AT&T maintains that this move saved $15 million (1 percent of its healthcare expenses) for all of 1993, its first year of operation. The percentage saved may be less for some plan sponsors or greater for others. It depends on the plan design and the current operating procedures between sponsor and administrator.

In addition to fewer claims paid for major medical policies, there are additional savings for those companies that offer pharmacy card programs. One large card processor (PCS) has determined that 5 percent of all pharmacy claims are paid for ineligible claimants because of the time lag between enrollment data becoming available to the employer and getting to the card processor.

Electronic Eligibility Reporting

The use of electronic enrollment data could provide additional savings if employers were to require their benefit administrators to support electronic eligibility reporting. Benefits are available to both healthcare providers and employers. Having electronic eligibility data available would enable providers to manage credit risk. In a world in which providers are uncertain about the amount of a final payment, that uncertainty results in credit losses that add to the cost of health care. Payers that can guarantee prompt payment to providers can obtain significant discounts. This is a win-win solution, but it requires accurate, up-to-date enrollment information as the foundation of accurate eligibility reporting.

Elimination of Duplicate Payments

Additional savings would be certain if duplicate payments stemming from overlapping coverage were eliminated. Since the 1980s, significant social change has made the old notion of "family coverage" obsolete. As more women have entered the work force, overlapping coverage has increased. Working couples often have individual coverage under their respective employers' plans and may cover each other as dependents as well. Children residing in the same household may have different sources of coverage: One child's health care could be the responsibility of an ex-spouse, whereas the other siblings are covered under their mother's or father's plan. Generally speaking, employees do not understand the rules that determine which plan pays first. They may submit claims to every available source of coverage and expect that carriers and administrators will work together to determine correct payments. That is not how the industry does business, and duplicate payments are the unfortunate result.

Until the data is collected electronically (a relatively inexpensive process), there is no way to measure the magnitude of duplicate payments. The solution is for employers in a region to share enrollment data, using a common database, and support an eligibility reporting mechanism. In this way, the coverage status of spouses, ex-spouses, and so on, could be kept current. Providers would have a source that would enable them to direct claims to the rightful payer, and in all likelihood they would be willing to pay for access to such eligibility information. Employers could be confident that they were not paying claims that should rightfully be paid by another employer. Considering how tightly organizations control the process of issuing purchase orders, comparable controls of the coordination of benefits process appear to be in order.

FURTHER APPLICATIONS OF EDI TO THE HR DEPARTMENT

EDI Payments to Benefit Administrators

Another major transaction flow from the HR department can be automated. EDI payments to all benefit administrators is the next step in the automation of the payroll and benefits process. Everyone is familiar with the payroll process. After time and attendance information is used to update the payroll system, the payroll program is run to create wage payments and related deductions. A great many wage payments are automated through direct deposits to employees' bank accounts. Deduction information is calculated for every pay period, but unlike wages, related monetary transfers may take place less frequently. Funds and information about benefits are transferred to benefit administrators as premiums or contributions. Premiums are paid for a variety of insurance products, including life insurance, worker's compensation, disability, and accidental death and dismemberment. These flows are illustrated in Figure 7–3. Retirement contributions are made for 401K investments and other savings plans. Payroll deduction information may be calculated by the company payroll program or by different vendors. In many companies, deduction information is printed and sent to the HR department. Periodically (quarterly, monthly, or more often), HR staff compile deduction information.

FIGURE 7–3
*A variety of insurance products require data and funds that an employer
can transmit electronically.*

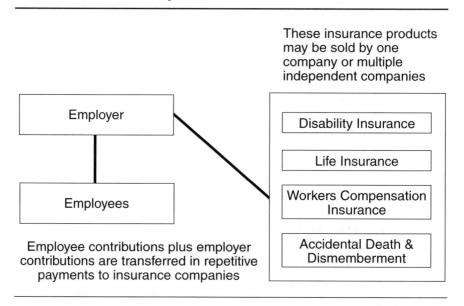

Because all this information is available in an electronic format,
the HR department can use EDI and electronic funds transfer
(EFT) to automate the movement of all of the funds and data gathered through payroll deductions. Steps have been taken to develop
the necessary EDI standards. For example, the ANSI X12 payment
standard, known as the Payment Order/Remittance Advice (820),
was amended to accommodate the needs of the pension industry.
This was necessary because an employee may elect that a deduction be split many ways, with portions of the deducted amount
being allocated to different investment funds. Funds can also be
allocated to the repayment of 401K loans.

Although electronic premium and pension payments may be
on the EDI frontier today, it is likely that they will be widely supported by payroll systems and processors by the end of this
decade. A natural evolution will occur as soon as HR managers
ask for EDI applications in their requests for system proposals.

Outcomes Research

By eliminating all redundant data entry, EDI can substantially reduce clerical data entry tasks. It can both save money through lower staffing levels and free the HR professional to focus on more important issues. The highest value-added task of the HR department is to fully use the most important asset of the organization: employee talent. The data capture process can obtain information that will provide additional insights for management. For example, managers are asking for "outcomes assessment" data, so that they can determine whether their healthcare-related expenses are really improving the health of their employees.

That assessment cannot come from provider data alone. Take the example of dental care. The American Dental Association suggests that a preventive dental health program can save significant lost time and prevent employee absenteeism. This hypothesis can only be tested by capturing absenteeism data and relating it to time absent for dental visits. Most time and attendance systems—even if automated with the latest magnetic card technology—are unable to provide qualitative data about lost time. HR professionals can use time and attendance collection to determine the *reasons* for lost time and relate them to the goals of a corporate wellness program. Although this is an electronic application, the benefits are not so much in the technology as in the insights obtained by the HR professional.

P A R T

III

IMPLEMENTING EDI IN HEALTHCARE SETTINGS

Chapter Eight

The Community Healthcare Information Network (CHIN) and Clinical EDI

During the late 1980s and early 1990s electronic standards and related software have evolved rapidly for both financial and administrative transactions in health care. In the mid- and late-1990s we can expect to see further expansion of EDI in the healthcare industry, but this expansion will have a change of direction. The emphasis will no longer be solely on administrative and financial transactions but will extend to clinical transactions. Clinical, financial, and administrative functions will be integrated into a seamless electronic network. As currently envisioned, such a network will form a community healthcare information network (CHIN) or some form of enterprise-sponsored healthcare information network (HIN). (See Chapter 3 for an introduction to these network types.) Although the CHIN will serve a provider/patient community, its components need not be within a local geographical area. The payer, reference laboratories, and other sophisticated clinical services may well lie outside the local area. In the world of EDI, no facility is electronically remote.

Two types of information will travel around the CHIN. Most financial and administrative functions comprise structured data that can be transmitted in standard electronic format. ANSI X12 standards have already been developed for many of these functions and more will follow. Clinical information, however, is unstructured and must currently be transmitted as freeform text in

E-mail. Current and future developments, however, will enable an increasing percentage of clinical information to be transmitted as structured data.

The CHIN will ultimately fulfill a variety of functions, including the following:

- Enhancement and expansion of applying EDI to financial and administrative functions
- The increasingly rapid exchange of data specific to managed care, such as requests for referral and referral authorizations
- Rapid and accurate communication of clinical data among physicians and other caregivers
- Archiving or "warehousing" of healthcare data
- Improved transmission of test requests and results
- Development of computer-based protocols to integrate the nursing staff into the healthcare team
- Collection of data necessary for utilization review and, eventually, outcomes research

ENHANCING FINANCIAL AND ADMINISTRATIVE FUNCTIONS

Healthcare industry managers should expect that the electronic data highways, currently used for claims traffic, will increasingly transport both financial and clinical information. These exchanges will not only be between payer and provider, but also among hospitals, physicians, laboratories, and allied health professionals.

The forces of change are being driven by two related developments: the progress in electronic claim processing and the computer-based medical record. The first transactions to be sent through a CHIN will be electronic financial transactions. Hospitals that are leaders in developing the organizational structure, the vendor relationships, and the trained personnel to do business electronically will undoubtedly be the first to link with other providers in the CHIN model. Often the healthcare financial manager, charged with making patient accounting decisions, is consciously or unconsciously determining the institution's overall network strategy.

Primary medical records are still usually paper-based. However, since 1987, the Health Level 7 (HL7) group (an organization of hospital system vendors and hospital information systems professionals) has been working on standards that can be used to move information from one hospital application program to another. (See Chapter 2.) The use of clinical EDI will not wait for the perfect computer-based medical record, so healthcare managers should first focus on the information that other providers most often ask for and exchange today. This information includes face sheet data, laboratory reports, operative reports, and discharge summaries. Standards for the transmission of most of this information are already available.

INCREASING THE RATE OF EXCHANGE OF MANAGED-CARE-RELATED TRANSACTIONS

Those who practice medicine where managed care is an important way of doing business may show greater interest in the managed care applications of EDI. A *request for authorization and authorization approval*, together with their respective reference numbers, could be exchanged both rapidly and accurately. Indeed, the computer exchange of data may go a long way to resolve the paradox that although managed care can reduce medical costs, the benefits are lessened by the increased workload for administering such care. It makes sense for both administrative and clinical information messages to be exchanged electronically.

Managed care companies that would like to automate the referral and utilization review process should consider working with physicians to support electronic clinical and administrative exchanges.

COMMUNICATING CLINICAL DATA AMONG PHYSICIANS AND OTHER CAREGIVERS

Many of the computers in today's medical offices or hospitals merely automate claims processing. Computers are still rarely seen in the consulting room, yet the physician who uses a computer system for recording and transmitting all, or part of, a medical record can enjoy substantial benefits. Computer-based medical records (CBMR) will result in rapid, accurate communication of clinical data among physicians and other caregivers. CBMRs have the potential for improving patient care, increasing efficiency, and slashing healthcare costs. The users of such systems—the physicians involved with patient care—need to have a vision of the potential of such an electronic medical record.

What can be done with an electronic patient medical record? The computer in the consulting room will link physicians through a network to other physicians, within a medical group or hospital or among physicians outside the facility. Computer-based medical records will be used in decision making.

REPLACING PAPER-BASED MEDICAL RECORDS

If the paper-based medical record were eliminated, shelves of dusty, dog-eared manila folders would be replaced by electronic storage of data for a computer program accessible by authorized inquirers, even by multiple authorized users at the same time. Consequently, the patient's medical record would always be available; it would never travel through the billing office, lie on someone else's desk, or be the subject of the oft-repeated response, "I am sorry, we can't find his records, doctor." In the medical office, "front office" staff would no longer need to spend valuable time "pulling" or searching for records.

Computer-based medical records will always be complete; even records from decades ago could easily be recalled using computer-based archives. Records will always be legible, nurses will always be able to read orders, and a physician will never again have to struggle with a vacationing colleague's handwriting. In fact, the old jokes about physicians' illegible handwriting will even become obsolete.

WHAT NETWORKS CAN DO FOR PHYSICIANS

Medline, the most widely used "external" networking service, enables physicians to access on-line databases for references in medical literature and pharmacological information, including adverse drug reactions and interactions. This, however, is just the first step in applying telecommunications to medical practice. The potential for using electronic networks is vastly greater than merely reading on-line reports. Here are some possibilities:

- Using network linkages, a physician could order laboratory tests, prescriptions, physical therapy, and other procedures or treatments.
- Test results could be inserted electronically into the patient's record.
- The receipt of urgent test results could be flagged by the appearance of a symbol or icon in a corner of the physician's computer screen.
- An additional benefit would be the "acknowledgment of receipt" for every order successfully delivered from the physician's computer. (Automatic acknowledgment of receipt is integral to the concept of EDI.)
- Acknowledgment of receipt of a prescription could be followed by confirmation that the prescription had been filled by the patient.

COMPUTER-BASED DECISION MAKING

Nothing is more likely to antagonize physicians than the idea that their hard-earned expertise might be replaced by a machine. Nonetheless, there are situations where most physicians, no matter what their prejudices, would agree that computer-aided decision making would be welcome. The first of these is the patient who has a multisystem disease that defies easy diagnosis. In this situation, information on the possible diagnoses, the probability of each possible diagnosis being correct, and the investigations most likely to yield an answer to the diagnostic dilemma could be obtained from a specifically designed database.

Computer-based decision making would also be helpful in emergency situations in which the decision-making process focuses less on diagnosis and more on "what to do next." An additional attractive use for computer-based decision making would be to integrate nursing staff more completely into the medical care team. In both emergency situations and routine office care, the physician could move between patients while a nurse progressively entered data into a computer and followed the instructions it indicated.

A great deal of routine office care could be delegated to the nurse practitioner who follows a computer-based protocol, leaving the physician free to deal with more complex medical problems.

COLLECTING DATA FOR UTILIZATION REVIEW AND OUTCOMES RESEARCH

In a CHIN the sponsor may be responsible for utilization review and outcomes research. A retrospective utilization review may ask the questions: "Did the physicians provide the most appropriate and cost-effective care?" and "Was referral to a specialist appropriate?" Outcomes research may ask a variety of questions, such as: "How well does one primary care physician manage patients with asthma compared with other physicians?" "Which inhaled corticosteroid gives the best results with the fewest side effects?" Obtaining data for outcomes research once meant conducting a laborious search through handwritten patient charts. In a fully electronic CHIN the data can be trapped and analyzed in a fraction of the time and at a fraction of the expense once required.

Both day-to-day medical service and retrospective outcomes measurement will be conducted better, faster, and cheaper through EDI and CHINs. The way that a CHIN functions and clinical EDI will work may best be understood by looking at the way a patient and the information about her condition move through the healthcare system.

CASE REPORT: THE CHIN IN ACTION

Suppose a patient named Janice has just started a new job with a large company by relocating to a new city. She is particularly glad that her company provides healthcare benefits, because her history of asthma has previously made it difficult for her to obtain healthcare insurance that has not excluded her asthma as a preexisting condition. Janice has had asthma and seasonal hayfever since childhood. At present, she is not taking any medication regularly but relies on an inhaler to relieve episodic asthma symptoms.

Her employer is a member in good standing of the local healthcare information network or CHIN and is therefore able to enroll

FIGURE 8–1
Enrollment transmitted from an employer to a payer.

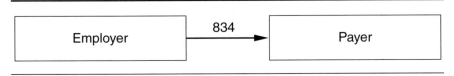

Janice in one of the company's health plans electronically. The plan that Janice chooses is a health maintenance organization in which her primary care physician is paid on a capitated basis, while "out of plan" services are paid on a fee-for-service basis. The X12 standard for enrollment is Benefit Enrollment and Maintenance (834) (see Figure 8–1). The payer sends back acknowledgment of Janice's enrollment electronically to her employer and Janice is relieved to know that her new healthcare benefits are effective immediately.

Emergency Room Visit and Follow-Up with Primary Care Physician

Several months later, Janice, who is enjoying the higher wages that result from her new job, moves from her small apartment to a larger one. As she packs her belongings, including her books, she experiences intensive exposure to dust. That night she has an asthma attack that is not relieved by using her inhaler, and by 11 PM she decides to go to the local emergency room.

While Janice is in the waiting and triage area, the hospital inquires electronically about her healthcare insurance eligibility using the X12 standard Health Care Eligibility/Benefit Inquiry (270) and promptly receives an electronic response confirming her eligibility and giving details of her coverage, using the X12 standard Health Care Eligibility/Benefit Inquiry (271) (see Figure 8–2). What a good thing she was enrolled electronically!

The emergency room physician determines that the asthma attack was precipitated by exposure to dust and treats her with a bronchodilator medication via a nebulizer machine. She responds well to a single treatment and is discharged after a period of observation.

FIGURE 8–2
Hospital Eligibility Inquiry (270) and Eligibility Response (271) to a payer.

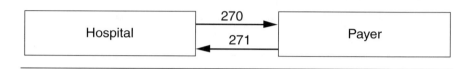

FIGURE 8–3
Hospital claim submitted using a Health Care Claim (837) as an encounter to a payer.

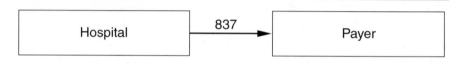

She is advised to use her asthma inhaler for any residual symptoms during the night and to contact her primary care physician the following morning.

The costs of her treatment—basic emergency room charge and excess time supplement—are keyed into a computer terminal in the emergency room. All supplies are barcoded and their costs recorded with a barcode reader. The physician's fees may be recorded separately. All this information is automatically uploaded to the hospital's mainframe computer. After Janice's discharge, the cost and service information is downloaded to a PC in the accounts receivable department, which transmits an electronic claim to her insurance plan for the ER services using the X12 standard Health Care Claim (837) as shown in Figure 8–3.

Simultaneously, the hospital computer uses the CHIN to advise Janice's primary care physician that the "encounter" has occurred. Figure 8–4 diagrams the process. This advice might be in the form of an E-mail message. However, structured EDI messages, using the X12 Health Care Service Review standard (278) will enable her physician's computer-based patient record to identify the correct

FIGURE 8–4

Health Care Services Review standard (278) used for a discharge summary sent by the hospital to the primary care physician.

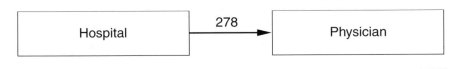

patient and place transmitted data in the appropriate portions of the record. The EDI message might communicate the following information:

> Janice Wells, social security number 157-48-3300, was admitted to the Community General Hospital ER at 11 PM on 3/4/96 suffering from a severe asthma attack. Lung function was 50% normal. She was treated with albuterol via nebulizer and responded well. After 1 hour her lung function was 75% normal. She was discharged with the advice to use her inhaler when necessary and to contact you today.

The next morning Janice calls her primary care physician and makes an appointment for later that day. The physician's front office initiates an electronic inquiry via the same CHIN and promptly receives an electronic response, using the same EDI (270/271) standards as the ER. (Refer again to Figure 8–2.)

When Janice sees her primary care physician she is feeling fine and her lung function is normal. The physician, however, discovers that Janice had an increase in the frequency of her asthma symptoms during the past year. He decides that she needs some medication on a regular basis to prevent asthma symptoms, so he prescribes an oral medication, theophylline, that she should take twice a day. Again using the CHIN, the prescription is sent electronically to Janice's regular pharmacist and an acknowledgment of the receipt of the prescription is returned. No X12 standard is available for this transaction as yet (see Figure 8–5).

The primary care physician has a capitated contract with the payer, so only an electronic record of the encounter needs to be sent to the insurance plan. Janice pays a $10 copayment for the office visit. In order to keep the HMO informed of the services rendered, an encounter report is transmitted by the physician (see Figure 8–6).

FIGURE 8–5
Prescription requests can be sent electronically from a physician to a pharmacy, but no X12 standard exists as of the mid-1990s for this exchange.

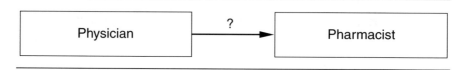

FIGURE 8–6
The physician informs the HMO of services rendered using a Health Care Claim (837) as an encounter report.

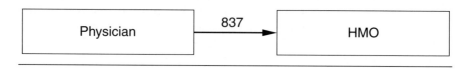

Specialist Referral

Several months later Janice again consults her primary care physician because her asthma seems to be getting worse and her medication isn't relieving the symptoms. On this occasion the primary care physician decides to refer her to an allergist for further evaluation. The primary care physician can authorize referrals and notify the payer so that the allergist's fee-for-service bill will be paid when submitted. Through the CHIN an electronic referral authorization is submitted to Janice's insurance plan. Referral authorization is accommodated by the X12 278 transaction set; patient information is accommodated by the Patient Information transaction set (275). Both are sent electronically to the allergist, as shown in Figure 8–7.

When Janice keeps her appointment with the allergist, the referral request and the referral authorization information have already been received by the allergist's office computer system. The correct reference numbers are already in the system; no eligibility inquiry

FIGURE 8–7
The physician authorizes a visit to a specialist, notifies the payer of the authorization, and transmits clinical information to the specialist for review before the patient arrives.

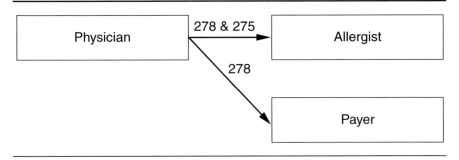

is necessary and no billing problems are anticipated. The specialist has already had the opportunity to review the clinical information in the referral request and is aware that Janice has been referred to her because the primary care physician is concerned about Janice's failure to respond to appropriate asthma treatment. Through the CHIN the specialist has the opportunity to obtain further clinical information about Janice from her primary care physician's records and her ER records, if she considers it necessary.

In taking Janice's history, the allergist learns that Janice was previously skin-tested for allergies five years ago when she lived in a different part of the country. After performing a physical examination and lung function tests, the allergist decides to repeat the skin-testing in case Janice has acquired some new allergies. Janice also mentions that on several recent occasions she has felt light-headed after eating foods containing peanuts and wonders if she could be allergic to them. Because severe allergic reactions can follow skin-testing to peanuts in symptomatic individuals, the doctor orders a blood test (RAST) for allergy to peanuts. The CHIN is used to transmit the order to the laboratory electronically and, in turn, the result will be received electronically (see Figure 8–8) (This laboratory report will never get lost!). Currently, there is an X12 Lab Report transaction set; but there are also lab report standards from the HL7 and ASTM organizations and which will be used has yet to be determined by the industry.

FIGURE 8–8

Laboratory test requests can be transmitted electronically, but the
industry has not indicated which standards will be used most often.

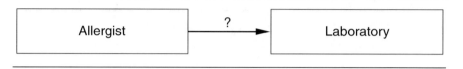

FIGURE 8–9

The allergist submits a claim (837) and the payer initiates an electronic
payment (835) for services rendered.

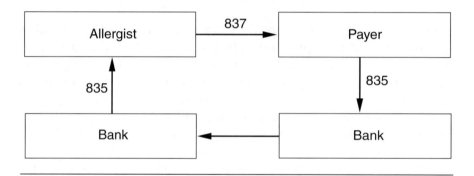

The skin tests show that Janice has indeed acquired some new
allergies and is highly sensitive to house dust. The allergist suggests that Janice continue to take her present medication but also
recommends the regular use of a corticosteroid inhaler to prevent
further asthma symptoms. As before, the prescription is transmitted directly to Janice's local pharmacist. The allergist also advises
Janice to take measures to avoid house dust exposure.

The allergist has a negotiated fee-for-service arrangement with
Janice's insurance plan. Consequently, her office staff submits an
electronic claim to the payer using the 837 standard.

To pay the invoice, an electronic remittance advice is sent to the
allergist using the 835 standard. Simultaneously, an electronic

FIGURE 8–10
The lab report, referral report, and lab payment can all be done electronically.

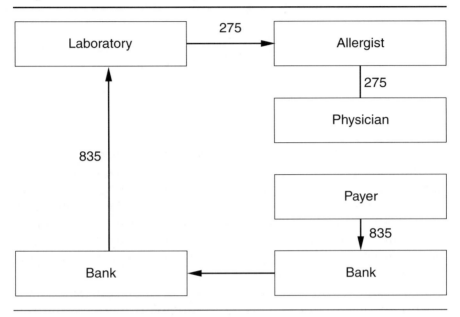

funds transfer (EFT) is sent to the provider's bank by the payer's bank, as shown in Figure 8–9. Janice pays only her usual copayment at the time of service by the allergist.

The allergist then reports her findings, evaluation, and recommendations for management to the primary care physician (electronically, of course!). The report of the laboratory test (it was negative for peanut allergy) is transmitted electronically not only to the allergist but also to the primary care physician. The Patient Information (275) standard may be used for these transactions. At her discretion, the allergist may transmit an addendum to her report, commenting on the significance of the result. A further loop of the CHIN allows the laboratory to submit an electronic claim for its services and receive an electronic remittance advice and EFT payment, as shown in Figure 8–10. (Janice's plan covers laboratory services in full, so she has no copayment.)

FIGURE 8–11
The hospital can request a paid claims file from a payer, but the standard for this process has not yet been designed or approved.

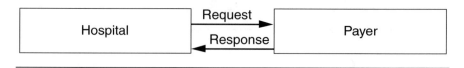

Recurrence of Asthma

Several months later, again after cleaning her apartment, Janice has another severe attack of asthma that does not respond to treatment with her inhaler. This time she remembers to call her primary care physician, who decides that she should go to the emergency room. While she is on her way to the hospital, Janice's physician transmits an electronic authorization for ER treatment (see Figure 8–7), avoiding the possibility that the payer will subsequently question the need for ER treatment.

When she reaches the ER, her demographic information is already available and her insurance eligibility verified. On this occasion she fails to respond satisfactorily to treatment and the ER physician decides to admit her under the care of her primary physician.

Once notified of this decision via the CHIN, Janice's primary care physician transmits his initial treatment orders to the hospital electronically. No X12 standard exists for this transaction, so the physician uses E-mail. By the time he arrives at the hospital, Janice's in-patient treatment is already under way and she is gradually responding. Once the physician has seen and examined Janice, he makes several alterations and additions to her existing treatment orders. Because he is concerned about this second ER visit and the slowness of her response to treatment, he asks the allergist (in the form of an electronic referral, shown in see Figure 8–7) to review her case the following morning at the hospital.

So that all pertinent clinical information is available to Janice's physicians, the hospital's medical record department requests all existing information that is available about Janice on the CHIN network (Figure 8–11) to place on her current electronic chart.

FIGURE 8–12
Allergist requests pharmaceutical claim data and the response reveals
lack of patient compliance with the daily medication regime.

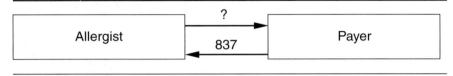

The allergist agrees that Janice's current treatment regimen should be adequate to control her asthma and suspects that inadequate compliance with prescribed medication may be an issue. On checking the result of a blood theophylline test that had been ordered at the time of admission by the primary care physician, the allergist finds that theophylline was not present in Janice's blood although she has been told that she should take this medication daily. The allergist then inquires via the CHIN for paid pharmaceutical claim data, asking specifically for the number of times Janice has filled her prescriptions for theophylline and the corticosteroid inhaler in the last four months (see Figure 8–12). The allergist calculates that it should be three to four times, but the payer can identify only one paid claim. No X12 transaction has been identified for this information exchange.

The allergist reports the data and her conclusion to the primary care physician. They agree to discuss the issue of compliance jointly with Janice. During the discussion, Janice admits that after one month's treatment she felt so well that she stopped taking her medication. The doctors explain to Janice the importance of continuing to take these medications on a regular basis. The allergist arranges for Janice to see her nurse who is experienced in patient education and enhancement of compliance. Janice is discharged from the hospital under the care of her primary care physician.

After Janice's discharge the hospital once again submits an electronic claim to the payer using data collected from various departments, including the emergency room. This information, as before, will have been collected by a combination of direct data entry and barcode readers. The primary care physician (who has a capitated agreement with the payer) needs to submit an electronic encounter advice, whereas the specialist (who has a fee-for-service contract with the payer) submits an itemized electronic claim.

Janice sees the allergy and asthma nurse several times and also calls her after discharge with questions. Janice gradually learns the way each of her medications works to control her asthma. Armed with this knowledge, Janice becomes progressively more compliant with her medication, and her asthma symptoms gradually disappear.

When Janice's primary care physician and her allergist meet at a hospital conference six months later, the primary care physician tells the allergist that he has just seen Janice on a routine office visit. He is delighted to report that she has been virtually symptom-free for five months and intends to remain so. In discussing Janice's case they both realize that they might have considered the issue of noncompliance earlier. In so doing, Janice might not have required hospital admission. They also appreciate, however, that her hospital admission has helped Janice understand the potential severity of her asthma. Consequently Janice has greater motivation for better compliance with her physicians' advice.

Conclusions about the Usefulness of the CHIN

By now a great deal of information about Janice has traveled along various pathways of the CHIN. It has helped to ensure the exchange of clinical, financial and administrative data in a timely, seamless, and error-free fashion. Janice's treatment has never been delayed because necessary information was not available, she has never had to pay more than the anticipated copayment or wait for months for reimbursement, and she has never been faced with an unexpected additional charge. Our patient is a happy camper!

Janice's physicians are also happy about the way the CHIN has worked for them. Again, clinical and financial data have always been in place when required, no test results have been mislaid, the primary care physician enjoys the freedom from the hassle of invoicing the payer, and the allergist appreciates the promptness with which her claims have been processed by the payer. These physicians now see the CHIN as the "way to go" for the future.

Chapter Nine

Organizing for EDI

In many ways, the nontechnical aspects of an EDI initiative can be more daunting than the technical issues surrounding EDI implementation, because the organizational issues fomented by EDI usually are more complex than the technical ones. Perhaps that is why estimates are that the human costs of education, training, and implementation management are 90 percent of the cost of doing EDI.

A SUGGESTED EDI
IMPLEMENTATION STRATEGY

In order to successfully implement EDI, a strategy is needed for organizing the process of change. The following steps to organizing are crucial in making EDI a reality.

Step One: Recognize the Need for Change

Most managers agree that doing business electronically and eliminating paper make sense. The fact is that today's organizations are organized to move paper. Every sizable company has a mailroom and a mailroom manager. But who, if anyone, is responsible for managing the electronic mailroom? Who will set the policies and procedures for security and confidentiality? Who will train the staff to understand that the "check is in the mail" no longer describes payments in an era of electronic funds transfer (EFT)?

How will projects such as receiving electronic invoices and electronic remittance advices be coordinated and prioritized? Who is in charge of making EDI the standard operating procedure? These changes and the related staffing needs can be met through an EDI organizational strategy and plan.

Step Two: Develop an EDI Organizational Strategy

The purpose of an organizational strategy is to structure the nontechnical requirements in your organization. This framework provides direction to all parties involved in the EDI initiative and fosters cooperation among the players. People requirements such as the EDI director (coordinator) and members of the EDI team, along with appropriate job positions and responsibilities, will be determined based on the framework. Personnel resources required for successful completion of tasks, types of tasks to be completed, and a realistic EDI timeframe with target dates for project completion will be developed.

Today's staffing requirements were designed for yesterday's technology. The managerial challenge of EDI is to design jobs for doing business tomorrow.

Step Three: Prepare a Mission Statement for EDI

The EDI mission statement should reflect the direction and commitment of the organization. The following general statement can be used as a starting point:

> We are committed to the use of standard ANSI ASC X12 and EDIFACT electronic transactions with our trading partners whenever possible. (Your name here!) desires EDI integration into everyday business practices to the extent that adding a new trading partner becomes a standard operating procedure. While the use of paper documents will continue for some time, those trading partners that wish to enjoy a long term relationship with our organization are advised to implement EDI capability as soon as practical. Trading partners that wish to do business electronically are advised to consult our manual entitled," A Guide to Doing Business Electronically" which contains a list of EDI standard transactions supported and the names of individuals to contact about EDI.

What is needed to support this statement?

- An EDI team with the resources and experience to help implement change
- An organization that understands what EDI and electronic commerce are and is ready, willing, and able to change

The organizational strategy must be designed to create the EDI team and to change how the organization does business. The mission statement sets the goals.

Step Four: Appoint an EDI Team

Dedicating staff may seem difficult with today's restrictions on hiring full-time employees. Nonetheless, most large organizations will need an EDI team whose initial full-time mission will be the low-cost implementation of new transaction sets and solicitation of additional trading partners. This team will first establish specific EDI policies and procedures created to meet the business challenges of your organization. They will then develop the EDI workplan for implementation.

The makeup of the EDI team is important. It is important that this team be considered more than "techies that eliminate paper." This team will be composed of "network enablers" who will achieve improved customer service and better business procedures for internal administration. The team should be seen as a business unit with technical support in the information systems (IS) department rather than an IS team. The blend of business people with IS people should reflect the necessary partnership during implementation of users and IS staffs. Integration of EDI messages into business operations changes people's jobs. Users must manage the automated workflow. User ownership of design and implementation is crucial.

What will the EDI team do? It will provide expert resources who can help users and the IS staff plan and implement EDI. The EDI team will provide experts who will participate in or direct transaction-specific projects. Those projects will require project management teams composed of user department representatives and IS staffers. EDI projects span multiple departments. They can

FIGURE 9–1

Proposed organizational relationships among IS, the EDI team, user groups, and the EDI steering committee.

EDI Steering Committee

Senior Management Champion
EDI Director
Information Systems
Finance
Claims
Materials Management/Purchasing
Legal, Audit, & Human Resources

IS Department	Finance Department	Claims Department
VP IS	VP Finance	VP Claims
Staff X,Y, Z	Representatives B1, B2, B3	Representatives A1, A2, A3

EDI Team
EDI Director
Staff 1, 2, 3

Project 837
Rep A1
Staff Z
Staff 3

Project 835
Rep A1
Staff Z
Staff 3
Rep B1

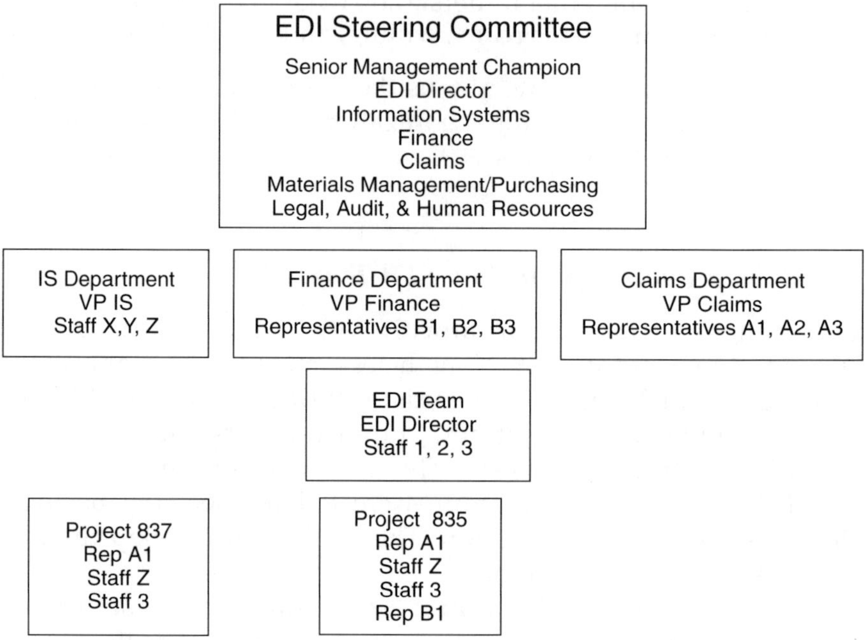

be coordinated through an interdepartmental EDI steering committee. The EDI team will be represented by their EDI director on that steering committee.

Figure 9–1 illustrates the organizational relationships that develop among EDI team members, staff, and the steering committee.

Example

How will the EDI steering committee, EDI team, and users work together? Implementation projects are often organized around the paper document that is to be replaced. For example, an 837 claims project group will meet to plan and implement the business and technological workplan design for a claim payer. The group is composed of three members (see Figure 9–1):

- *A representative from the claims department* (to lend perspective on the business needs of the trading partners)
- *A representative from the IS department* (to lend expertise in the technological requirements and EDI implementation resources)
- *A representative from the EDI team*—a member working in conjunction with the EDI director to provide additional direction and focus for the group in terms of the larger construct—the big picture—of the organization-wide EDI initiative

The EDI director will sit on the EDI steering committee along with representatives from the various user groups and provide the direction and leadership for the organization's EDI initiative.

Step Five: Appoint an EDI Director

The team just described will need a leader who is respected by management and combines business understanding, diplomatic skills, and an appreciation of data management and IS. Managing organizational change will be a critical skill as well the ability to deal with trading partners.

By way of illustration, James Whicker of Intermountain Health Care, Inc., was selected by management as director of EDI for the 24-hospital system headquartered in Salt Lake City, Utah. During a restructuring phase at Intermountain Health Care, an opening at the corporate office became available. Senior management determined that by moving the EDI timetable forward, the organization could move Mr. Whicker into the director of EDI position and provide a more focused, working relationship with the payers. Although Mr. Whicker finds his IS background helpful in this current position, his skills in communications and problem-solving expertise have been a major asset to the EDI initiative.

For example, Mr. Whicker determined there was a need for routine monthly meetings with local payers. These are payers he identifies as "those who already recognize the value of EDI." He now schedules an "EDI day" once a month to meet with representatives from Medicare, Medicaid, Blue Cross Blue Shield, HMOs/PPOs, and other companies starting new projects, to provide an open forum for communications with payers. He states, "This effort has significantly improved working relationships with payers. Together we prioritize projects, jointly identify problems, and work together to resolve them."

The development of an EDI education agenda should be part of the EDI director's job description. The role of the EDI director is to chair the EDI steering committee, working with representatives from multiple departments that will be affected by EDI. With input from this group and assistance from appropriate outside resources, the director of EDI will also guide the educational process.

Step Six: Allocate Resources to the EDI Initiative

In order for an ongoing commitment to the EDI initiative to take place, the necessary funds and resources must be generated and dedicated to the EDI mission. There must be funding for a realistic number of persons to oversee and implement the EDI initiative. It is crucial that the necessary funding and staffing be in place in order to ensure its success.

Funding should be considered for the initiation and completion of a comprehensive Trading Partner EDI Capable Survey. Survey results will serve three important roles in the EDI initiative:

- Provide the foundation for developing an EDI strategy by providing concrete data regarding the capabilities and needs of all of the trading partners
- Serve as the baseline for a trading partner profile database
- Communicate to all trading partners your commitment to an EDI strategy.

Step Seven: Obtain Senior Management Support

The communication of an EDI vision must start with senior management consensus. Consensus will create a clear, common focus for the adoption of electronic commerce. Management must create an atmosphere of employment security needed to overcome concern that automation is a euphemism for layoffs. Clear benchmarks and objective measurements of progress must be identified. To move from the existing paper processes to a paperless operation will take time and hard work. Realistic evaluations of progress are important to justify funding and maintain momentum.

The organization's EDI initiative will have a higher degree of success if the EDI strategic plan is supported by senior management. A lack of support by senior management will undermine the EDI initiative. Conversely, the ripple effects of an endorsement from senior management will provide the seal of approval. Project participants will be confident that, with senior management approval, the EDI initiative will be considered a vital component of the organization's vision.

Step Eight: Adopt an EDI Strategy and Plan

Once the EDI team is selected and in place, several immediate tasks need to be undertaken. First, the team should develop EDI policies and procedures consistent with the organization's overall corporate strategy. The EDI plan will be based on these policies and established activities, and these policies should be based on the vision expressed by senior management and the EDI director. General consensus among team members on the direction of the group and the scope of activities to be undertaken by the EDI team should be agreed upon by all.

To achieve the goals of the team requires significant coordination of efforts across multiple departments and systems. Coordination of EDI activities is required for all aspects of the technical work and business operations, both inside and external to the organization. The best way to ensure the coordination of activities and a successful EDI implementation is to develop a detailed EDI implementation workplan. This workplan identifies the tasks associated with the goals for EDI implementation. The workplan also includes timetables for completing tasks and identifies the persons responsible for carrying out each activity. If more than one person or department is involved in a particular activity, this will be noted in the workplan.

Step Nine: Implement EDI Education

In order to affect significant change within an organization, it is vitally important to conduct internal education. The purpose of the education is twofold:

- To create an understanding of the scheduled change and its process
- To justify the need for a new course of action

People affected by change need to know the nature of the change, how it will occur, its impact, and their role in the process. People do not object to change as much as they object to being changed. Their participation, buy-in, and active assistance are all the desired ends of the EDI educational program.

It is important for executives, managers, and personnel to understand EDI and its purpose and benefits, methods of operation, and the positive impact EDI will have on the organization's business. This is often one of the most difficult tasks to oversee and is accomplished in four steps:

1. *Tailor instruction appropriate to staff and management to include the basic elements of electronic data interchange and more advanced/technical levels of EDI education.* EDI education must be tailored to specific departments within the organization. Course material with electronic purchase order examples should not be used to teach patient accounting staffs when they will be dealing with electronic claims.

2. *Motivate organization members to recognize EDI as a way to conduct business more effectively.* Case study material from healthcare leaders can play an important motivational role. If benchmarking is part of the organization's culture, include EDI benchmarking studies. Explicitly relate EDI to the quality goals.

3. *Help members understand the impact the EDI process will have on existing business operations.* Healthcare managers can adopt radically aggressive goals for EDI implementation today that were not achievable three years ago. Hospitals can automate all of their Medicare remittance processing and eliminate half of their invoices and check payments.

4. *Move people to accept the business process changes that accompany EDI.* EDI can eliminate jobs, but concern about lost jobs can seriously hamper implementation. The EDI organizational strategy has to deal with the natural human reaction to the threat of job loss. How many organizations have more talented capable people than they need? As EDI eliminates the

work that once tied up dozens of administrative workers, the challenge should be to find other productive uses for good people.

THE ESSENCE OF ORGANIZING AN EDI IMPLEMENTATION

Ideally, a concerted effort should be made to integrate the technological and organizational strategies of the corporation. EDI operations are particularly sensitive to this need. The EDI initiative will be shaped by both strategies. Both an organization's information systems and human resource strategies must accommodate the transition to EDI and electronic commerce. With a balance between the technical and human resource elements, success is more than likely.

Chapter Ten

Financial EDI

Banking has been an integral part of the movement to EDI. During the last 15 years the financial services industry has been transformed by electronics. Automatic teller machines are ubiquitous. Most financial instruments—treasury notes and bonds, corporate debt, and stock certificates—are now in electronic "book entry" form rather than printed on paper. Corporate America has applied EDI to the payment process and has developed standards for EDI payments using electronic funds transfers (EFTs). In addition to standards for payments, EDI standards exist for other information exchanged with banks, as shown in Figure 10–1. These transaction standards fall into the general category of *financial EDI*, the electronic exchange of information between banks and their customers. Financial EDI standards are developed in the ANSI ASC X12 organization as are standards for insurance and material management.

ELECTRONIC FUNDS TRANSFERS AND FINANCIAL EDI

In 1991, an ANSI ASC X12 standard for the electronic payment of healthcare claims was approved. Because the standard has been mandated by the Health Care Financing Administration it is being adopted widely. By 1994, for example, every hospital in California had abandoned the use of paper remittance advices and checks for electronic Part A Medicare payments. This leadership by HCFA has opened the door for the widespread use of EFT and financial EDI by claims payers and healthcare providers. Treasury professionals at insurance companies and other benefit administrators, as well

FIGURE 10–1
Summary of financial EDI transaction standards.

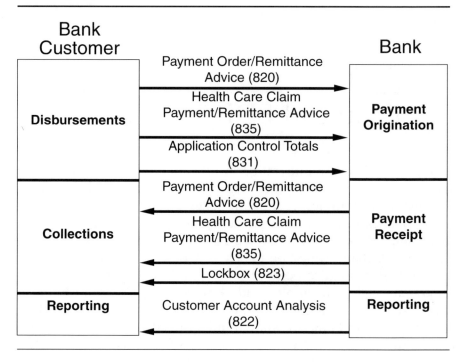

as those at provider organizations, need to know how electronic payments work. They also need to know how to work with EDI-capable banks to realize the opportunities afforded by financial EDI and EFT.

When Is Money Electronic?

Any discussion of EFT has to begin with a review of what money is and how it moves between payer and payee. Most people's understanding of how money moves in the banking system is not helped by descriptions from the popular press. Money is "wired," "traded," and "laundered." Descriptions of the international money market would lead the uninformed to believe that plane loads of dollar bills are being flown from one foreign capital to another. In fact, only a small fraction of money is currency.

FIGURE 10–2
Example of a paper check deposit transaction.

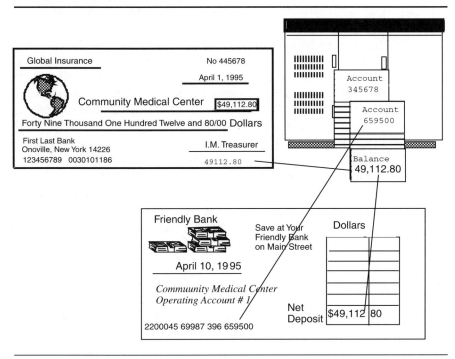

Bank deposits vastly exceed the amount of currency actually printed. This means that most funds are in fact electronic, consisting of deposit records maintained on computers at banks. This has been the case since the bank ledger cards on which deposits were recorded were replaced by computers.

Most "money" consists of computerized credit balances at banks, but people's instructions to banks about moving funds are usually given with paper documents.

Some of the confusion about EFT arises from a misunderstanding about how funds move among banks. A deposit transaction example as shown in Figure 10–2 illustrates the documents a provider uses to process a check from a payer. The process is as follows:

1. After a check is endorsed, it is deposited by the provider into its bank. The bank is able to identify the correct bank account to credit by means of a number on the deposit ticket furnished by the provider.

2. The amount to be credited to the account has to be keyed or encoded by a clerk and printed on the deposit ticket check in magnetic ink character recognition (MICR) characters so that the data can be read by a scanning device later in the process. The dollar amount also must be printed with MICR characters on the bottom right-hand side of the check.

3. Once the check and deposit ticket have been encoded, they are processed through a reader/sorter machine that captures the machine-readable data.

4. The "deposit proofing " process verifies that the total deposit equals the sum of the individual items. If the numbers are valid and check totals equal the deposit total, the appropriate bank account will be credited.

The Check Clearing System

The reader/sorter also capture the other MICR characters on the bottom of the check. This is the identification number of the bank on which the check is drawn, known as the *American Bankers Association (ABA) number.* These numbers are also referred to as *transit routing numbers.* They help banking institutions process checks received. Checks are sorted by the machine into separate "pockets" where checks drawn on a bank or banks in a particular geographical area are segregated. From that point there are multiple alternatives for collecting the funds:

*   The provider's bank can "present" the check to the payer's bank in a direct send presentment. This task, known as check clearing , appears mind-boggling. More than 12,000 U.S. banks and 2,500 savings and loans and savings banks can take deposits. Every bank has mechanisms in place to send checks to whatever bank is identified via the ABA number. Because more than 55 billion checks are routed through the banking system each year, there are armies of messengers and fleets of cars, trucks, and planes moving checks among banks all over the country.

- The bank may send the check to a clearinghouse, where bank representatives gather to exchange checks. Clearinghouses have been used for hundreds of years in major money centers such as New York and London.
- The bank may send the check to a large correspondent bank, which processes checks for smaller banks.
- The bank may give the check to its Federal Reserve Bank for collection.

The role of the Federal Reserve System in both check payment and electronic payment mechanisms is important and worth a short review. Although most nations have one central bank, the United States has the Federal Reserve System comprising 12 Federal Reserve Banks. All depository institutions such as commercial banks, savings banks, and savings and loans have a deposit account with a Federal Reserve Bank. The Federal Reserve System operates a check clearing mechanism available to all depository institutions that maintain accounts with it. The Fed, as it is called, also acts as the final settlement bank in the check collection process as each day's check clearings are totaled and obligations between banks are settled. The check clearing process operates with many rules and many different deadlines that govern daily "settlement" procedures and affect the availability of funds. The payer's check would be only one of many checks exchanged between two local banks.

In order to illustrate the flows, the example shown in Figure 10–3 assumes that the provider's bank (Friendly Bank) gives the Global Insurance Company's bank (First Last Bank) checks totaling $1,049,000. On the same day, First Last Bank also gives Friendly bank $1,000,000 in checks drawn on it. A net settlement amount of $49,000 is owed to First Last Bank by Friendly Bank. In this example, the net settlement is made by a transfer of $49,000 on the books of the Federal Reserve Bank where both banks maintain accounts.

The ability of one bank or depository institution to credit another does not require both to hold accounts at the same Federal Reserve Bank. The computers at each Federal Reserve Bank are connected via an electronic network that can carry payment instructions among all the Federal Reserve Banks. This allows a bank in one part of the country to instruct its Federal Reserve Bank

FIGURE 10–3
The settlement function of the Federal Reserve Bank in interbank payments.

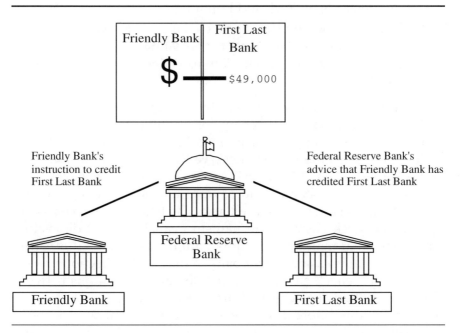

to debit its account and credit the account of a depository institution, with an account in the Federal Reserve System, in another part of the country. Moving funds electronically between Federal Reserve Banks is fundamentally different from moving funds using checks because there is no paper.

Wire Transfer Payments

Wire transfer is the fastest way to move money, because it transfers funds among banks on the same day within minutes after instructions are given by the originating bank to its Federal Reserve Bank. Wire transfers are done through the Federal Reserve System and are also called *Fedwires.* As was the case with a paper check payment, money is always transferred by means of a credit to one electronic ledger and a debit from another. For a Fedwire payment the instructions pass among different banks via a telecommunications link.

Unfortunately, in common parlance this transaction would be described by saying the money was "wired," as if funds were physically sent over some form of electronic cabling. The difference between paper checks and EFTs is not whether the money is "electronic" but whether the interbank payment mechanism is paper-based or electronic. Payers that use the Fedwire are initiating on-line payments. A major difference between a Fedwire payment and all other payments is that Fedwires transfer "good funds" or nonreturnable items, resulting in what is called same-day availability of funds.

The Fedwire transactions carrying the credit initiation message from the payer's bank also transmit a small amount of information to the payee's bank for the account of the payee. This information identifies the payer and provides some remittance detail related to the payment. Fedwires are the most expensive payment mechanism and may cost $15 to $40. Fedwire users can reduce their cost by initiating Fedwires using a computer terminal or PC instead of telephone or written instructions.

Automated Clearinghouse (ACH) Payments

An automated clearinghouse (ACH) payment is an electronic file that contains much of the information found on a paper check in a standard format developed and maintained by the National Automated Clearing House Association (NACHA). NACHA is an association of regional automated clearinghouses. The development of the ACH network was pioneered in California in the 1970s, but its broad usage nationally owes a great deal to its adoption by the Social Security Administration, which currently makes 41 million payments a month through the ACH network.

As the banking system adopted computers the traditional exchange of bags of checks was replaced when practical by electronic media. Rather than exchanging bags of checks at the local clearinghouse, banks gradually migrated to exchanging computer tapes. Regional automated clearinghouses act as modern counterparts to their paper-check-orientated predecessors. ACH payments are exchanged electronically between banks, and a net settlement amount for each day's electronic presentments is exchanged on the day after ACH items are exchanged. For this reason, ACH payments are referred to as next-day items. ACHs exchange payment information among themselves, and net settlement is made through the Federal Reserve System. In contrast to Fedwire payments, ACH payments provide a low-cost method of electronic payment.

ACH payments have different formats for different types of payments. In addition, NACHA rules allow X12 formatted remittance data to move through the ACH network along with electronic funds. As a result, ACH payments can contain more remittance information than Fedwires do and as much remittance detail as accompanies most checks. Some of the most commonly used NACHA formats are as follows:

- *Cash concentration and disbursement (CCD),* used by many businesses for intracompany transfers such as the movement of funds from multiple branches or stores with deposits in local banks to a central corporate depository account. The CCD has no room for administrative information, so its usefulness as an intercompany payment is limited.

- *Cash concentration and disbursement plus addendum (CCD+),* used by the federal government to pay its vendors. The CCD+ format has one feature not shared with the CCD: the ability to send up to 80 characters of information, which can be in an ANSI X12 format. An ANSI X12 Trace number segment is designed to be transmitted in the CCD+ 80-character record. Because this format can combine both data and dollars it is well suited to make intercompany payments.

- *Prearranged payment and deposit (PPD),* used extensively to make direct deposits of employee payroll payments, deposit social security payments, and collect insurance premiums from individuals. The PPD format is used for consumer payment transactions only.

- *Corporate trade exchange (CTX)* , in which large amounts of information, such as remittance detail, accompanies funds through the ACH. The CTX format was designed to transport ANSI X12 payment data within the ACH network.

There are two X12 payment standards. The Payment Order/Remittance Advice (820) is a general payment mechanism used by providers to pay vendors. The Health Care Claim Payment/Advice (835) is specifically designed to accommodate remittance detail for healthcare claim payments. The 820 and 835 are identical except for the remittance detail area of the 835, which was expressly designed for the remittance details associated with the payment of healthcare claims. Both allow the originator of a payment to send remittance detail either separately or with electronic funds.

Any ACH payment format can be used for either debits or credits. A credit transfer might be initiated by an insurance company for credit to the account of a healthcare provider or by a healthcare provider to pay a supplier. A debit transfer might be used by an insurance company to collect premiums from individual customers, whereas a healthcare provider might initiate debits to collect funds from patients for the self-pay portion of their medical bill. Because each type of payment yields different benefits, most providers and payers will send or receive some combination of checks, Fedwires, and ACH payments as their needs dictate.

Electronic Payments and Float

Financial managers in different areas of responsibility view payments differently:

- Cash managers tend to focus on when and how money moves because of the impact of float on funds available for investment.
- Controllers and accounting managers tend to focus on the who and why of payments, and are concerned with remittance detail related to the funds received.

The concerns of cash managers, controllers, and accounting managers can all be met by EDI payments. The first issue that always arises in any discussion of electronic payments is that of float. Electronic payment is frequently erroneously equated with faster payment by payers and payees alike. However, payments need not be made faster just because they are electronic. Electronic payment describes *how* payments are made, not *when*. Electronic payers and payees alike have more control over disbursement/collection timing than do those who use checks. They can precisely determine when funds are to be transferred.

In fact, the experience with EFT in the corporate sector often indicates that electronic payments do not result in faster payments. The largest users of corporate payments have made the transition to electronic payments in a "float-neutral" way, by making the timing of disbursement of electronic funds equivalent to the timing of receipt of "good funds" when checks are used. For example, if check payments were mailed 30 days after receipt of an invoice and funds are cleared to the vendor's account on the 33rd day, electronic payments can be scheduled to arrive on the 33rd day as well. Float is a matter to be discussed and negotiated but should never be a deterrent to using electronic payments.

Electronic Remittance Information

EDI payments involve more than EFT. The issues of electronic remittance information must also be addressed. This chapter has dealt with the different payment mechanisms, including the electronic transfer of funds through the banking system. Nonetheless, the process of payment involves more than the movement of money. Because payment involves both treasury and accounting, it is best understood as a process and not as a transaction. The payment process combines the transfer of funds and related remittance activity. Payment requires the exchange of information from the payer's accounts payable program to the payee's accounts receivable program as well as the transfer of funds from the payer's bank account to the payee's bank account. An EDI payment requires the electronic transfer of remittance information from the payer to the payee together with the transfer of electronic funds from the payer's bank account to the account of the payee.

Like other EDI transactions, this exchange of data and funds should be accomplished by using computer-processable data in a standardized format, without human intervention. Because the payment process involves the transfer of both information and money, it is somewhat more complicated than are other EDI transactions. Most EDI transactions are bilateral: They occur between

FIGURE 10–4
*Payers can make funds transfers and send remittance data through
banks. Some payers also use VANs to move remittance data.*

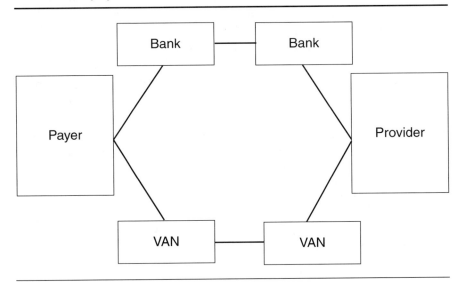

two trading partners. EDI payments on the other hand, require at
least four parties to the transaction: the payer, the payer's bank,
the payee, and the payee's bank. They may also involve a value
added network.

Although trading partners can exchange EDI messages across a
variety of electronic networks, they can only move funds through
the banking system. Electronic payments differ from paper payments, which seldom separate checks and remittance information
sent to a payee. Some payers send funds through the electronic
banking network and remittance information through another
separate nonbank network. The major value added networks
(such as GEIS, MCI, AT&T, Advantis, and Sterling Software) that
transport such EDI transactions as purchase orders also transport
EDI remittance data. Because they are not banks they cannot move
funds through EFT.

Figure 10–4 illustrates the options open to a claim payer, who
can send electronic remittance data through the banking system

either with electronic funds or separately. Similar options are available to providers making EDI vendor payments.

In a paper-based environment, checks are usually attached to remittance advices. When remittances are processed, usually a clerk visually confirms that the dollar amount on the check matches the dollar amount on the remittance. If a payer decides to transmit electronic funds through the banking system and remittance data through another network, the question arises as to how the payee is to reassociate banking records with accounting data. Procedures must be installed by the payee to confirm that payment has been received before receivables are posted and closed.

Any organization that implements an EDI payment system has two broad options, which contain many minor variations:

- Send or receive both dollars and related remittance data through the banking system.
- Send or receive dollars through the banking system and remittance data through another electronic network.

In the EDI literature, this is known as the "dollars and data" issue. Different circumstances dictate the use of one option or the other. If dollars and remittance data are separated, the payer creates the additional task of reconcilement or reassociation for the payee. Using a trace number to link the EFT with the related remittance data is the best procedure when the payer does not use the banking system for the remittance information. EDI creates a new set of service requirements for bankers and new opportunities for financial managers concerned with bank services.

Until recently most financial managers have not had any reason to think of the banking system as an electronic information network. Nonetheless, that role is inevitable; the conversion from paper checks to EFT requires it. Electronic funds cannot be used for electronic payments without electronic information to identify the payment. The consideration of data reporting issues represents a new responsibility for the treasury management function. In the past, treasury and banking functions were self-contained and isolated in finance. The use of EDI payments requires the treasury staff to consider systems issues. To make EDI payments, a financial manager must evaluate the adequacy of the data in the accounts payable application program. To receive EDI payments, the treasury staff must obtain information needed in the accounting department in addition to the information needed for cash management.

The use of EDI payments also changes the nature of the bank services required. If financial managers are going to link with the electronic bank information network, their banks have to do far more than mail statements once a month. This is well understood by the banking community. Within NACHA, bankers have formed the Bankers EDI Council to act as a forum for banks that want to provide EDI services to their customers. In order to educate bank customers and other bankers, the council publishes guidelines that can help providers determine whether their banks are "EDI capable."

Not all banks have invested in the software and telecommunications capability necessary to meet providers' EDI needs. They are unlikely to do so until their customers ask for such services or threaten to move their accounts to those banks that do support financial EDI. In order to aid those treasury managers who want to assess their banks' EDI services, the Bankers EDI Council has developed an EDI-Capable Questionnaire, reprinted in Appendix B of this book.

THE COLLECTION PROCESS

The Funds Collection Process Today

The funds collection process today includes the receipt of mail and such cashiering tasks as reconciling the amount of a check with remittance detail, preparing deposit tickets, and delivering checks to the bank. Many organizations use bank lockboxes to handle their deposits. A *lockbox* is a post office box from which checks are picked up by a bank's courier service. Lockboxes are used to reduce the float of mailed checks and accelerate the collection of funds. Checks taken from the post office in the early hours of the morning can be endorsed, deposited, and routed for collection before the organization would normally have received those checks in its daily mail delivery from the postal service.

In addition to accelerating the collection of investable funds, a lockbox service can perform some data entry tasks, such as MICR encoding and the capture of limited remittance details for electronic transmission to the provider. Most providers that use lockboxes arrange for remittance paperwork to be forwarded to their patient accounts departments. Lockbox systems date from innovations of the late 1960s. Unfortunately, many lockbox processes have gained little in efficiency in recent years. Costs continue to include redundant rekeying tasks and the transportation of paper checks all over the country.

The Funds Collection Process Tomorrow

Widespread use of EFT and EDI for claims payments is imminent, so it is important for financial managers to consider the consequences. First, existing lockbox arrangements have been designed to minimize mail float. When checks are no longer coming by mail, such arrangements will be partially or completely obsolete. For larger providers, the location of the lockbox should be reevaluated and possibly shifted as some claims payers convert to EFT.

In all likelihood, some claim payers will opt to use the banking system for the transmission of remittance data, but others will not. When payments and remittance data are sent separately, providers will need information from their receiving banks that will enable them to reconcile incoming electronic credits with numerous remittance advices sent through other electronic networks. If EFT payments do not include enough data to match the payment to remittance information sent under separate cover, the provider will inherit the difficult and time-consuming task of reassociation.

To prevent this situation the EDI standard for healthcare remittance information was designed to assist in the process of reassociation. An ANSI X12 segment called TRN or Trace can be included in the remittance data and in the EFT. Because the CCD+ format contains an 80-character addendum record that can hold the TRN segment, providers should work with a bank that can capture the CCD+ addendum record and transmit it with a confirmation of the funds deposited. On receipt, the provider can automatically reconcile payment information with remittance detail.

Financial managers also have the choice of receiving remittance detail through the banking system, although only a portion of the nation's banks support this option. Some managers want to receive dollars and data together, but these payees should be aware that it may make sense to receive remittance data electronically from some payers before funds are transferred. Early receipt of remittance data can speed the generation of claims to secondary payers, thus accelerating cash flow. Some Medicare fiscal intermediaries provide this service.

Financial managers will have to develop a strategy for how they wish to be paid. Receiving the desired payment format will require the assistance of others in the organization, particularly the individuals who negotiate payer contracts, to ensure that trading partners are informed about how to make payments. Providers will also have to cope with a variety of paper and electronic payments, and their banks will have to collect funds in multiple formats and report collection information as best suits the providers' needs. The EDI-capable bank should be a partner in connecting payers and providers in a "seamless" payment process that avoids human intervention.

THE DISBURSEMENT PROCESS

Why adopt electronic payments? During the budgetary approval cycle, financial managers have to present cost-benefit analyses about proposed expenditures, and a proposal to automate disbursements can expect to encounter objections to the merits of the investment. The benefits of originating EDI payments are substantial, but they can be lost in a sterile debate about why an organization should spend the money to replace checks with EFTs. Eliminating the check is not the goal of EDI payments. The replacement of the check with its electronic counterpart is the least significant benefit of using EDI payments. The benefits of originating EDI payments come from other aspects of automating financial operations. For claims payers, EDI and EFT can be used to improve all the communications between plan sponsors, employees, and providers. For healthcare providers, electronic vendor payments should be part of an overall EDI strategy to automate all transactions in the procurement process.

The Disbursement Process Today

Benefit administrators generally issue payments from a claim adjudication system, whereas healthcare providers generally issue payments from an accounts payable system. With the advent of capitation contracting many providers become claims payers and face the same challenges faced by benefit administrators. The disbursement issues of payments generated by accounts payable and claim adjudication systems will be addressed.

Disbursement from Accounts Payable Systems

Payment occurs at the end of the purchase cycle, and it is affected by the accounts payable approval process. The accounts payable department in most provider operations is facing an ever larger number of invoices because of changing material management practices. As the materials management department has shifted warehousing responsibilities from internal staff to outside distributors, the number of invoices has increased. Those providers considering "stockless purchasing" should pause to consider what will happen when the volume of invoices more than triples from their principal distributors alone. The financial consequences of an overloaded accounts payable department can be significant. Available discounts are frequently not taken. Shortcuts include approving invoice prices just to move the paperwork, even if the purchase order price is lower. All too often providers negotiate attractive group purchase contracts, but the desired reduction in supply costs is lost in the accounts payable department.

The accounts payable process involves matching receiving documents, invoices, purchase orders, and subsequent authorization for payment. The payment process begins when an entry to the accounts payable system authorizes payment. Most systems can schedule payments according to terms kept resident in the vendor file (the computer profile of each vendor). Providers print checks at different intervals and the payables program generates checks and related remittance advices for each vendor, if those payments are scheduled for release during that print cycle. Printed checks are frequently reviewed by the payables staff against the original documents, and there are different check review procedures depending on the monetary amount of the payment.

The timing of payments and the control requirements for payment release are issues that will continue to be addressed after electronic payments are adopted. What providers should consider seriously is the complete elimination of payment by check. The time-consuming process of check printing and mailing involves drudgery work for many talented people and is not much more streamlined today than 20 years ago.

There are a number of inefficiencies:

- The check printing process involves a limited production run on a check printer used as seldom as once a week.
- Check stock is expensive and represents a security risk that must be accommodated by appropriate security procedures.
- Check printing may involve spoiling several checks in order to correctly align the printer. Updating the check register file and procedures related to check reconcilement is a related expense.

The payables systems that process this ever-increasing number of transactions are frequently among the oldest application programs in the provider organization. Some are limited in their ability to reference more than a few invoice numbers per remittance advice. Thus, some hospitals that are pioneering "just-in-time" delivery procedures require the distributor to process hundreds of checks and remittance advices per month.

ELIMINATING CHECKS THROUGH THE USE OF ELECTRONIC PAYMENTS

As mentioned earlier, EDI payment involves the transfer of remittance information from the accounts payable program of the payer to the accounts receivable program of the payee. It also involves EFTs from the payer to the payee. EDI payments should be considered for use with suppliers that will provide electronic invoices in a reciprocal exchange. Providers should encourage suppliers to send electronic invoices in return for electronic payments.

Originating Electronic Vendor Payments

Most of the information used to generate an EDI payment resides in the accounts payable system. Providers must determine whether the information generated by the accounts payable program and printed on the remittance advice is accurate and complete. The required detail for making an EDI payment is found in the EDI standard known as the Payment Order/Remittance Advice (820). Although most accounts payable programs provide some payment detail, some information will undoubtedly be lacking. There has been no reason before the use of EFT to maintain the bank account number of the vendor and the American Bankers Association (ABA) identification number of the vendor's bank. That information is needed to complete an electronic payment to the vendor. There is also a need for an indicator to flag certain payments made via checks and others through EFT.

Providers face the same options about sending remittance data and dollars separately or together that have to be addressed by the claims payers. Providers may choose to direct some vendor payments through the ACH network (data and dollars together). In that case, an EDI Payment Order/Remittance Advice (820) is converted by the provider's bank to the CTX format so that remittance data can be sent through the banking system. Providers might also choose to send vendor payments through a bank and remittance data through an additional network (data and dollars apart). In that case an EDI Payment Order/Remittance Advice (820) is converted by the provider's bank to a CCD+ format with an appropriate trace number and the remittance data is sent through a network other than the banking system.

The need to generate payments requires the services of EDI-capable banks. An EDI-capable disbursement bank should be able to accept a computer file of payment orders (820s) from a provider and convert them to the appropriate payment format. The EDI-capable bank should provide a variety of methods to handle payment origination, including reformatting files into NACHA payment formats as needed.

ADDITIONAL AUTOMATION OPPORTUNITIES

Providers may choose to automate trade payments to vendors because of the importance of the relationship with key vendors and the tie to receiving electronic invoices. Then providers can move to a broader plan to eliminate check payments. The broader plan should deal with two different payment recipients: employees and vendors that are not major trading partners.

Employee Payments

When providers review their check volume, they discover that many items are generated for travel and entertainment expenses or reimbursements to employees for subscriptions or similar expenditures. Employee reimbursement is an important transaction flow to automate via EFT. Many corporations have attacked this expensive reimbursement process in several ways, but the result is eliminating checks and directly depositing reimbursements into the employees' accounts. This step may eliminate as much as 25 percent of total check volume. The savings available from automation of employee reimbursement stem from reduced paperwork in the accounts payable department and higher employee productivity.

Direct deposit of employees' payroll checks has been adopted by most corporations during the last 20 years because it eliminated the longer lunch hour taken by employees to go to the bank to cash their paycheck. Unfortunately, employees now receive checks from flexible spending administrators and from benefit administrators as well as checks for reimbursement of travel and entertainment expenses. All these payments may necessitate that same trip to the bank that direct deposits were designed to eliminate. The key to direct deposit of healthcare reimbursement checks is giving the benefit administrator the appropriate account number for each employee. That can be done using the 834 Benefit Enrollment and Maintenance transaction set standard.

Other Vendors

Although automating payments to key suppliers can eliminate tens of thousands of transactions, some providers report that 80 percent of their purchases account for only 2 percent of their expenditures. Vast numbers of small purchases are done with contracts and purchase orders. As was described in Chapter 6, checks for these purchases can be eliminated using corporate procurement cards. Purchases made using cards are paid for by one payment to the provider's merchant card bank. This reengineering of the procurement process can have a dramatic impact on the total number of checks eliminated.

Disbursement from Claims Adjudication Systems

The potential for saving money from the automation of payments by benefit administrators is quite significant. The EDI standard for the payment of healthcare claims is the Healthcare Claim Payment/Advice (835), which was approved in 1991. This standard can initiate a funds transfer and transmit an explanation of benefit/remittance advice.

Healthcare claims generate enormous numbers of checks and related explanations of benefit (EOB) and remittance advices. Many benefit administrators produce one check and EOB for a provider, one check and EOB for the employee, and one EOB for the employer, all as a consequence of a single medical encounter! Although some insurance companies can "bundle" claims payments made to one provider and reference multiple claims, there are many benefit administrators who cannot. This is because they administer claims for many self-insured companies and do not want to commingle funds among the different plan sponsors. Claim payers who want to adopt EDI and EFT face some of the same shortcomings in their claims adjudication systems as are exhibited by accounts payable systems also designed without EDI and EFT capabilities. There is a need to capture provider and employee bank account numbers and the transit routing numbers of their banks. In addition the system must indicate which payees want to be paid electronically and how they wish to receive their funds and data electronically.

The task of changing from the check and EOB printing process to an EDI and EFT payment process can be daunting to the financial managers of benefit administrators. As is the case for providers contemplating conversion to EDI payments, the case for conversion should not be made on a comparison of check costs versus EFT costs. The adoption of EDI payments is a part of an automation strategy applied to the entire claim process. Benefit administrators who adopt electronic claims payments will leverage the efficiencies they enjoy from electronic claims receipt. The movement to EDI and EFT can precipitate a reengineering of the treasury functions, the adoption of EFT debits to fund employer disbursement accounts, and the use of laser check printing to replace impact printers. As is the case with other companies moving to EDI payments, the overall process improvement and relationship improvement opportunities are far more important than the savings of an electronic funds transfer versus a check.

Outsourcing Check Printing: Completely Paperless Payments

Providers and benefit administrators may start to convert payments to electronic transfers, but for some interim period they will have to support both EFTs and check payments. There is an alternative that manages both processes simultaneously. Financial managers can consider outsourcing the check printing and mailing function.[1] Banks and other vendors offer the service of receiving an electronic file and converting the information to printed checks and remittance advices that are then mailed. EDI-capable trading partners receive EDI payments under this system. Organizations that outsource their check printing can immediately convert to a paperless payments system.

Outsourcing is not an option for all financial managers. However, it should be considered by those that would like to streamline their operations and not support dual (paper and electronic) disbursement procedures.

---

[1] "Payables Efficiency Measurements Send Processing to Banks," *Corporate Cashflow*, October 1992, p. 11.

APPENDIXES

APPENDIXES

Appendix A

Bibliography

PERIODICALS

"Automated Medical Payments News" is a newsletter published by Faulkner and Gray, 118 South Clinton, Suite 700, Chicago, Illinois (312-648-0261).

"Corporate EFT Report," "EDI News," and "Electronic Messaging News" are newsletters published by Phillips Publishing, Inc., 7811 Montrose Road, Potomac, Maryland 20854 (800-777-5006).

EDI Forum is a good source for in-depth articles about international EDI, EDI standards development, the history of EDI, and other professional commentary. Reading back issues of this journal may be one of the best ways to learn about the field's development and growth. Published by the EDI Group Ltd., 221 Lake Street, Oak Park, Illinois 60302 (708-848-0135).

EDI World is a monthly publication that provides as inexpensive introduction to current developments in EDI. Published by EDI World, 221 Coolidge Street, Hollywood, Florida 33020-2012 (305-925-5900). *EDI World* has published several special issues dedicated to healthcare EDI.

"Health Data Management" is also available from Faulkner and Gray, 118 South Clinton, Suite 700, Chicago, Illinois (312-648-0261).

Healthcare Financial Management, although not dedicated to EDI, has produced more in-depth articles about EDI from the provider's perspective than has any other professional journal. *HFM* is published by the Healthcare Financial Management Association, Two Westbrook Center, Suite 700, Westchester, Illinois 60153 (800-252-4362).

BOOKS

Baum, Michael S., and Henry J. Perritt, Jr. *Electronic Contracting, Publishing, and EDI Law.* New York: John Wiley & Sons, 1991. 871 pages.

Bort, Richard, and Gerald R. Bielfeldt. *The Handbook of EDI.* Boston: Warren Gorham and Lamont, 1994.

Emmelhainz, Margaret A. *Electronic Data Interchange: A Total Management Guide.* New York: Van Nostrand Reinhold, 1990. 256 pages.

Kimberley, Paul. *Electronic Data Interchange.* New York: McGraw-Hill, 1991.

Wright, Benjamin. *The Law of Electronic Commerce.* Boston: Little Brown and Company, 1991. 432 pages.

Appendix B

EDI-Capable Questionnaire

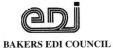
BAKERS EDI COUNCIL

Treasury Management Association
Formerly NCCMA

RECEIPT

1. Indicate which of the following EDI/EFT formats your bank is currently capable of receiving:

   ☐ A. CCD
   ☐ B. CCD+
   ☐ C. CTP
   ☐ D. CTX
   ☐ E. ASC X12 820 (from the originating entity or a VAN)
   ☐ F. Other (please specify)

2. Indicate which format translations your bank provides for delivery of remittance data.

Output Formats

BAI	ASC X12 820	823	Proprietary	Other	Payment Formats Received
☐	☐	☐	☐	☐	CCD
☐	☐	☐	☐	☐	CCD+
☐	☐	☐	☐	☐	CTP
☐	☐	☐	☐	☐	CTX
☐	☐	☐	☐	☐	ASC X12 820
☐	☐	☐	☐	☐	Fedwire
☐	☐	☐	☐	☐	Check
☐	☐	☐	☐	☐	Other

3. For incoming payments, indicate your bank's ability to deliver associated remittance detail into the output media indicated.

Payment Formats

CCD+	CTP	CTX	ASC X12 820	Other	Output Media
☐	☐	☐	☐	☐	Terminal/PC
☐	☐	☐	☐	☐	Paper
☐	☐	☐	☐	☐	Diskette
☐	☐	☐	☐	☐	Mag Tape
☐	☐	☐	☐	☐	CPU to CPU*
☐	☐	☐	☐	☐	VAN

*Mainframe or personal computer

4. Indicate, if for reporting purposes, Fedwire, ACH and lock-box can be combined into a single report format or a single data transaction. Please describe the formats and output media you support for this process.

5. Indicate what information your bank can report on incoming payments through your bank's information reporting system: (attach sample reports if appropriate)

   ☐ A. Detailed information on payments and amounts only

   ☐ B. Detailed information on remittance information

6. A. Indicate whether your bank can report electronic payment information on a same day or next day basis and via what methods:

Same Day	Next Day	Output Media
☐	☐	Information reporting
☐	☐	Paper
☐	☐	Diskette
☐	☐	Mag tape
☐	☐	CPU to CPU*
☐	☐	VAN

*Mainframe or personal computer

B. Indicate what time the information is made available to receivers.

7. Please indicate other ASC X12 financial transactions sets your bank supports:
   - ☐ A. 821 – Financial Information Reporting
   - ☐ B. 822 – Customer Account Analysis
   - ☐ C. 823 – Lockbox
   - ☐ D. 828 – Debit Authorization
   - ☐ E. Other

8. Discuss your bank's support for debit receipt services.

ORGANIZATION

1. Indicate which formats your bank can accept to originate payments:
   - ☐ A. ASC X12 820
   - ☐ B. CCD
   - ☐ C. CCD+
   - ☐ D. CTP
   - ☐ E. CTX
   - ☐ F. Other (please specify)

2. If your bank can accept payments in the ASC X12 820 Payment Order/Remittance Advice indicate which types of payments your bank can create:

Remittance Detail/Data Format (Output)

ASC X12 820	CCD+	CTP	CTX	Fedwire	Check	EDIFACT	Payment Types
☐	☐	☐	☐	☐	☐	☐	CCD+
☐	☐	☐	☐	☐	☐	☐	CTP
☐	☐	☐	☐	☐	☐	☐	CTX
☐	☐	☐	☐	☐	☐	☐	ASC X12 820
☐	☐	☐	☐	☐	☐	☐	Proprietary format
☐	☐	☐	☐	☐	☐	☐	Other

3. Indicate the capabilities your bank has for accepting payment instructions from your customer using the following input media.

Payment Formats

CCD	CCD+	CTP	CTX	ASC X12 820	Input Media
☐	☐	☐	☐	☐	Diskette delivered to the bank
☐	☐	☐	☐	☐	Magnetic tape delivered to the bank
☐	☐	☐	☐	☐	CPU to CPU
☐	☐	☐	☐	☐	Customer inputs using bank supplied personal computer software
☐	☐	☐	☐	☐	VAN mailbox
☐	☐	☐	☐	☐	PC Upload/On-line system
☐	☐	☐	☐	☐	Other (Describe)

4. A. Indicate the method(s) of transmission security your bank currently supports:

	PC	VAN	CPU	Other
Data Encryption	☐	☐	☐	☐
Message Authentication	☐	☐	☐	☐
Automatic Call/Dial Back	☐	☐	☐	☐
Other	☐	☐	☐	☐

B. Describe your hardware and/or software requirements for each feature/option:

5. Given an ASC X12 820 Payment Order/Remittance Advice file received from your customer, indicate whether your bank performs a syntax edit to ensure correct syntax. Indicate how long after the file is received such editing is performed.

6. Describe the types of ASC X12\Acknowledgment\Control transactions that your bank supports.
   - ☐   997 – Functional Acknowledgment
   - ☐   824 – Application Advice
   - ☐   831 – Control Totals
   - ☐   Other

7. A. Describe your bank's ability to warehouse ASC X12 820 advices.

   B. Indicate any time cutoffs for accepting transmissions prior to the creation and release of payments based on type.

   C. Indicate time frames for deleting/cancelling payments prior to the creation and release into the payment systems.

8. Describe any edits your bank's ACH system performs at the file and batch levels.

INDEX

Index

About the Authors

James J. Moynihan is a Principal in McLure, Moynihan, Inc., a firm offering consulting and research services, education, and implementation assistance related to Electronic Data Interchange applications for benefit administrators and healthcare providers. McLure, Moynihan, Inc., EDI healthcare research services, strategic plan consulting, and practical implementation assistance to claims payers, providers and professional associations. Mr. Moynihan has been active in the EDI standards movement since 1989, the year work first began on X12 insurance standards. He was the co-chair of the ANSI X12 insurance subcommittee's Payments Work Group that developed the first EDI standard for health insurance. Mr. Moynihan is the author of *The Implementation Manual for the Healthcare Claim Payment/Advice (835)*. His articles on health care and insurance EDI have appeared in numerous publications, including, *Health Systems Review, EDI World, Employee Benefits Journal, Healthcare Informatics, Journal of the AHMA, Corporate Cash Flow Magazine, EDI Forum, Managed Care Quarterly*, and *Healthcare Financial Management*. Mr. Moynihan received his bachelor's degree from Fairfield University and his M.B.A. from Rutgers University.

Marcia L. McLure, Ph.D., M.B.A. is a Principal in McLure, Moynihan, Inc. She is a member of ANSI ASC X12 and co-chair of the X12 Healthcare Transactions Steering Workgroup. Her articles on EDI have appeared in *EDI Forum, Healthcare Financial Management, Healthcare Interchange Report Magazine* and *EDI World*. Dr. McLure earned her BS degree from Loyola University of the South, New Orleans, her MS degree from the University of Missouri-Kansas City, and her Ph.D. degree from UCLA in research evaluation with a focus on management and policy.

Other books of interest to you from Irwin Professional Publishing...

THE HEALTHCARE SYSTEMS PLANNING MANUAL

Evaluating, Selecting and Implementing Information Systems Throughout the Organization

Geoffrey H. Wold and Robert F. Shriver

ISBN: 1-55738-604-8

THE DISASTER RECOVERY PLANNING MANUAL

Assessing Risks and Developing a Comprehensive Plan for the Healthcare Organization

Geoffrey H. Wold and Robert F. Shriver

ISBN: 1-55738-602-1

COMPUTERIZED HEALTHCARE INFORMATION

Developing Electronic Patient Information Systems

Michael W. Davis

ISBN: 1-55738-609-9

Also available in fine bookstores and libraries everywhere.